Nursing Care

In

Nuclear Medicine

The Complete Guide

ALEXANDRE CAREWELL

Table of contents

« Nuclear medicine: where patients literally light up from the inside so doctors can see what's wrong. »

Introduction

Nuclear medicine : a brief presentation.

Nuclear medicine, often shrouded in a veil of mystery due to its evocative name, is in fact a fascinating medical speciality that combines science, technology and care. It was born out of the encounter between advances in nuclear physics and medicine's constant need for new methods of diagnosis and treatment.

At the heart of this discipline are radiopharmaceuticals, radioactive substances used either to establish detailed images of the human body's internal processes or to treat certain diseases. What makes these substances special is their ability to target specific areas of the body, giving doctors an intimate and precise view of what's going on inside the patient, often well before symptoms appear.

In other words, nuclear medicine is a bit like having super-powerful eyes that can see beyond the surface, revealing details that other imaging methods cannot. This specificity makes it an invaluable tool for diagnosing pathologies such as cancer, heart disease and neurological disorders.

But nuclear medicine does not stop at diagnosis. It also plays a therapeutic role. Diseases such as certain types of thyroid cancer are treated by using radioactivity to target and destroy the diseased cells, an approach that has revolutionised the treatment of these patients.

Behind this cutting-edge technology, however, there is a profoundly human dimension. Every procedure, every scan, every treatment involves a patient with his or her worries, hopes and needs. And this is where collaboration between healthcare professionals, including nurses specialising in nuclear medicine, is essential. They are the link between complex technology and the patient, ensuring that every step is carried out with care, compassion and expertise.

So, beyond isotopes and scans, nuclear medicine is a story of continuous innovation in the service of humanity, a field where science and care meet to bring hope to many patients around the world.

The central role of the nurse.

Nurses are much more than mere cogs in the medical machinery; they play a central role in the care of nuclear medicine patients. Their role goes far beyond the administration of care; it also encompasses the patient-caregiver relationship, the coordination of treatments and the role of educator.

Firstly, it is essential to understand that the nurse is often the first point of contact for the patient. Before a scan is carried out or a treatment administered, it is the nurse who welcomes, reassures and prepares the patient. In a world where radioactivity is often synonymous with anxiety or fear, the nurse's ability to inform and instil confidence is vital.

The humanity of nurses is also evident in their role as educators. They are not just there to administer medicines or monitor equipment. They also explain procedures, answer questions and demystify fears. In so doing, nurses give patients the keys to becoming active players in their own care.

In nuclear medicine, nurses also play an essential technical role. Preparing radiopharmaceuticals, monitoring patients during examinations, managing potential side effects: all these tasks require specialised expertise. The nurse is the guarantor of patient safety in an environment where precision and vigilance are essential.

But beyond these technical responsibilities, the nuclear medicine nurse is also a coordinator. They are the link between the doctor, the technician, the patient and sometimes other health professionals. Their role is to ensure that everything runs smoothly, that information flows and that each stage of the medical process is optimised for the patient's well-being.

If nuclear medicine is a complex symphony of technology, science and care, the nurse is the conductor. They ensure that every note is played to perfection, and that the patient, at the centre of this melody, receives the best possible care with compassion, skill and dedication.

Chapter 1:
FOUNDATIONS
NUCLEAR MEDICINE

History and development
of nuclear medicine.

Nuclear medicine, a discipline at the crossroads of physics, biology and medicine, has a rich history that reflects the rapid development of technology and knowledge over the course of the 20th century.

The history of nuclear medicine began in earnest with Henri Becquerel's discovery of radioactivity in 1896, followed shortly afterwards by Marie and Pierre Curie's work on radium and polonium. These discoveries laid the foundations for understanding the properties of radioactive materials and their potential medical uses.

In the 1930s and 1940s, with the development of the first cyclotrons, it became possible to produce radioactive isotopes artificially. These instruments opened the door to the use of radioactive substances to visualise and treat diseases. The first successful treatment of a thyroid condition using radioactive iodine in 1941 marked a turning point.

The post-war period saw a rapid expansion of nuclear medicine, supported by advances in technology and investment in nuclear research. In the 1950s, the concept of scintigraphy was introduced. This technique uses special cameras to detect the radiation emitted by radioactive isotopes introduced into the body, making it possible to visualise the distribution of these isotopes and diagnose a variety of pathologies.

The 1970s saw the arrival of positron emission tomography (PET), a major advance that provides three-dimensional images of the human body with unprecedented resolution. Coupled later with computed tomography (CT), this technology became an invaluable tool for diagnosing and monitoring many diseases, particularly cancers.

In the late 20th and early 21st centuries, nuclear medicine continues to evolve with the advent of new imaging techniques, new radiopharmaceuticals and more targeted treatments. Image fusion, such as the PET/CT combination, offers better localisation of lesions and more complete information.

Today, nuclear medicine is a well-established speciality, recognised for its ability to provide unique insights into the physiology and pathology of the human body. It is an example of how innovation, science and medicine can work together to transform patient care and offer new perspectives on diagnosis and treatment.

Radioactive isotopes : friend or foe?

Radioactive isotopes, omnipresent in the world of nuclear medicine, often arouse ambivalent feelings. Their very name evokes both revolutionary medical advances and potential threats. Yet, like so many tools in the vast arsenal of science, these isotopes are neither intrinsically good nor inherently bad. Their value lies in the way we use them.

Friends in diagnosis and treatment
The beneficial potential of radioactive isotopes in medicine is indisputable. They are essential in the diagnosis of many conditions. Scintigraphy, for example, relies on the administration of radioactive isotopes to the patient to

obtain detailed images of the body. Once introduced, these isotopes are directed at specific organs or tissues, enabling doctors to detect abnormalities with unequalled precision.

What's more, some isotopes have the power to treat diseases. Cancers, for example, can be targeted and treated using radioisotopes. Their radioactivity destroys the diseased cells, offering an alternative or complement to other treatments such as surgery or chemotherapy.

Potential enemies if poorly managed
Radioactivity, however, is not without risks. Excessive or unnecessary exposure to radiation can damage healthy cells, increasing the risk of cancer or other conditions. That's why the amount and type of isotope, as well as the duration of exposure, are carefully calculated and monitored during every medical procedure.

In addition, the management of radioactive waste is crucial. Materials used in nuclear medicine must be stored, handled and disposed of with the utmost care to avoid contamination.

Valuable tools with great responsibility
Like any powerful scientific breakthrough, radioactive isotopes come with their share of promises and precautions. They symbolise the delicate balance between the potential for healing and the need for careful handling.

So radioactive isotopes can be both our friends and our enemies, depending on how we understand and use them. In the capable hands of nuclear medicine professionals, they are invaluable life-saving tools. But they also remind us of the serious responsibility that comes with the power of science.

Equipment: scintigraphy, PET, gamma cameras and more.

Nuclear medicine relies on a wide range of cutting-edge equipment to explore the human body non-invasively and to treat certain pathologies. Here is an overview of these machines, which are as fascinating as they are essential.

1. Scintigraphy :
Scintigraphy is a medical imaging technique that uses radioisotopes that are injected, inhaled or ingested by the patient. These isotopes emit gamma rays which are then captured by a gamma camera.

> Gamma cameras :
> This equipment detects the gamma radiation emitted by the radiopharmaceutical in the patient's body. They are made up of special crystals that transform the radiation into light, which is then converted into electrical signals to create images. The images obtained provide functional rather than anatomical information, showing how organs and tissues function in real time.

2. Positron Emission Tomography (PET) :
PET is a more advanced medical imaging technique than traditional scintigraphy. It uses isotopes that emit positrons. When these positrons encounter electrons in the body, they produce gamma rays which are then detected by the PET camera.

> PET camera :
> It resembles a CT scan and is often used in conjunction with it (PET/CT). PET images show where glucose is used in the body, which is particularly useful for locating tumours, which often consume more glucose than normal tissue.

3. Computer tomography (CT) :

Although CT is not specific to nuclear medicine, it is often used in combination with PET to obtain both anatomical and functional images. CT uses X-rays to create detailed images of the body.

4. Radiation therapy :
In addition to imaging equipment, nuclear medicine uses devices to administer therapeutic radiopharmaceuticals. These treatments can be administered in the form of injections, capsules or specific internal devices.

5. Protection and measurement systems :
Given the radioactive nature of the substances used, protective equipment such as lead shields, special gowns and dosimeters (which measure radiation exposure) are essential to ensure the safety of patients and healthcare professionals.
Over the years, the technology behind this equipment has evolved considerably, offering better image resolution, reduced radiation doses and more precise information about the human body. These advances continue to transform the way diseases are diagnosed, monitored and treated, making nuclear medicine a dynamic and essential part of the modern medical landscape.

The link between radiopharmacy and nuclear medicine.

Radiopharmacy and nuclear medicine are intimately linked, forming an inseparable tandem in today's medical landscape. To understand this close relationship, we need to define each field and examine how they intersect.

1. Radiopharmacy :

Radiopharmacy concerns the design, manufacture and dispensing of radiopharmaceuticals. A radiopharmaceutical is a preparation containing a radioactive isotope bound to a specific molecule or compound. These preparations can bind to specific tissues, organs or cells in the body, making it possible to visualise or treat particular conditions.

2. Nuclear medicine:

Nuclear medicine is a medical speciality that uses radiopharmaceuticals for diagnostic or therapeutic purposes. It can provide information on the function and structure of tissues and organs, or enable targeted treatment of certain diseases.

The link between the two:

Diagnosis :

Radiopharmaceuticals are used as contrast agents in nuclear medicine. When introduced into the body, they emit radiation that can be detected by equipment such as gamma cameras or PET scanners. These functional images reveal how organs and tissues function, and can detect abnormalities.

Therapy :

Some radiopharmaceuticals have therapeutic properties. For example, radioactive iodine can be used to treat thyroid disorders. In this context, the role of radiopharmaceuticals is to provide a safe and effective radiopharmaceutical to specifically target diseased cells or tissues.

Research & Development :

Radiopharmacy plays a crucial role in the search for new radiopharmaceuticals. This collaborative work with nuclear medicine enables us to innovate, improve diagnostic accuracy and develop new treatments.

Quality & Safety:

The production and dispensing of radiopharmaceuticals require strict quality standards to guarantee their efficacy and safety. Radiopharmacy professionals ensure that these standards are met, guaranteeing that the products used in nuclear medicine are both safe and appropriate.

Radiopharmacy and nuclear medicine are two facets of the same field, working hand in hand to improve patient care. The former provides the tools, while the latter uses them to diagnose and treat. Together, they embody the promise of precision medicine, focused on the individual needs of patients.

Chapter 2:
THE DAY-TO-DAY LIFE OF A NURSE IN NUCLEAR MEDICINE

Preparing the patient : before, during and after the exam.

Patient preparation is a crucial aspect of nuclear medicine. It guarantees not only the quality of the images obtained but also the safety and well-being of the patient. A nuclear medicine examination often requires specific preparation, which differs depending on the type of examination and the radiopharmaceutical used. Here is an overview of patient preparation before, during and after a nuclear medicine examination.

Before the exam :

- **Medical consultation:** Before any examination, patients should generally consult their nuclear medicine physician to discuss the purpose of the examination, their medical history, any medication they are taking and other relevant factors.
- **Fasting:** Some examinations, such as PET, may require the patient to fast for several hours before the radiopharmaceutical is administered.
- **Hydration:** It is often advisable to drink plenty of water before the examination to facilitate elimination of the radiopharmaceutical after the examination.
- **Comfortable clothing: We** recommend that you wear comfortable clothing and remove all jewellery or metal objects.
- **Specific instructions:** Depending on the examination, special instructions may be given, such as avoiding certain medicines or following a specific diet.

During the exam :

Administration of the radiopharmaceutical: The radiopharmaceutical is administered by injection, inhalation or ingestion. The patient may sometimes feel a slight sensation of cold or heat when injected.

Waiting time : After administration, it may be necessary to wait for the radiopharmaceutical to disperse in the body and reach the target organ or tissue.

Positioning: The patient is placed on an examination table, and it is essential to remain still during image acquisition to ensure image quality.

Communication: Throughout the examination, the medical staff will communicate with the patient, providing instructions and ensuring his or her comfort.

After the exam :

Hydration: It is often advisable to drink plenty of water after the examination to help eliminate the radiopharmaceutical from the body quickly.

Waiting for results: The images obtained will be analysed by the nuclear medicine physician, and the results will generally be discussed at a subsequent consultation.

Post-examination instructions: In rare cases, specific instructions may be given, such as avoiding close contact with young children or pregnant women for a short period, due to residual radioactivity.

Side effects: Side effects from nuclear medicine examinations are rare. However, if patients experience any discomfort or unusual symptoms after the examination, they should contact their doctor.

Patient preparation in nuclear medicine is essential for obtaining high-quality images, while ensuring patient safety and comfort. Good communication between the patient and the medical staff is essential to ensure that the examination runs smoothly.

Administration radiopharmaceuticals.

The administration of radiopharmaceuticals is a fundamental stage in nuclear medicine, requiring rigour, precision and compliance with protocols. Once administered to the patient, these radioactive substances are used to obtain diagnostic images or for therapeutic purposes. Let's look at this process in detail.

1. Types of radiopharmaceuticals :
There are many different radiopharmaceuticals, each targeting a specific organ, tissue or physiological process. The choice of radiopharmaceutical depends on the examination or treatment planned.

2. Route of administration :
- **Intravenous injection: The** most common method. The radiopharmaceutical is injected directly into a vein, usually in the arm.
- **Ingestion:** Some examinations, such as those of the thyroid gland, may require the ingestion of a capsule or liquid solution containing the radiopharmaceutical.
- **Inhalation:** For lung examinations, the patient may have to inhale a radioactive gas or aerosol.
- **Intra-arterial or intrathecal injection:** For specific procedures, the radiopharmaceutical can be administered directly into an artery or into the subarachnoid space around the spinal cord.

3. Preparing the patient :
Before administration, it is essential to check the patient's identity, confirm the examination prescribed and ensure that all pre-examination instructions have been followed. Allergies, current medication and relevant medical history should also be checked.

4. Dosage :

The dosage of the radiopharmaceutical is carefully calculated according to the examination, the patient's weight and other factors. The aim is to use the minimum amount necessary to obtain quality images while guaranteeing patient safety.

5. Safety measures :

Staff administering radiopharmaceuticals take protective measures to minimise radiation exposure, such as using shielded syringes, wearing gloves and using lead shields.

6. Patient monitoring :

After administration, the patient is sometimes monitored to ensure that there are no immediate adverse reactions. Although rare, allergic reactions or other adverse reactions may occur.

7. Disposal :

Radiopharmaceuticals are eliminated naturally from the body, mainly via the urinary tract. Patients are often encouraged to drink plenty of water after the examination to speed up this process. Precautions may be recommended to avoid radioactive contamination, such as washing hands after using the toilet.

The administration of radiopharmaceuticals is a complex procedure that requires specialist training, appropriate equipment and strict adherence to protocols. When carried out correctly, it provides valuable information for the diagnosis and treatment of many diseases.

Surveillance and security measures.

Nuclear medicine, although beneficial, involves risks associated with the use of radioactive substances.

Consequently, monitoring and safety measures are essential to protect patients, medical staff and the environment.

1. Patient protection :

Minimum dosage: Radiopharmaceuticals are administered in the minimum quantities necessary to obtain quality images or a therapeutic effect, while minimising exposure to radiation.

Patient information : Patients are informed of the risks and benefits of the examination or treatment. They are also given instructions on how to reduce exposure to those around them, if necessary.

2. Protection of medical staff :

Training: Staff are trained in the principles of radiation protection, safe administration techniques and emergency procedures.

Protective equipment: Gloves, lead aprons, protective screens and other devices are used to reduce exposure to radiation.

Dosimetric monitors: Staff wear dosimeters that measure their exposure to radiation over a given period.

Work protocols: Procedures are designed to minimise exposure time and maximise distance from radioactive sources.

3. Hygiene measures :

Hand washing: Rigorous hygiene is essential to avoid contamination.

Safe disposal: All radioactive waste, whether syringes, gloves or excretion products, is handled with care and disposed of in accordance with regulations.

4. Installation safety :

Zoning: Areas where radioactive substances are handled or stored are clearly identified and restricted.

Ventilation: Work areas are equipped with suitable ventilation systems to prevent the spread of radioactive substances.

Radiation detectors: Alarms and detectors are in place to signal high levels of radiation or leaks.

5. Environmental monitoring :

Regular monitoring: Radiation levels are regularly monitored in and around the facilities to ensure that they remain within acceptable limits.

Waste management: Radioactive waste is stored, handled and disposed of in accordance with regulatory guidelines, ensuring long-term safety.

6. Emergency plan :

Training and simulations: Staff are trained to respond to emergencies, and simulations are organised on a regular basis.

Response kit: Response kits for spills and other incidents are available and contain everything you need to manage an emergency situation.

Safety in nuclear medicine is an absolute priority. Thanks to strict regulations, in-depth training and appropriate equipment, the risks associated with the use of radioactive substances are managed and minimised, ensuring everyone's safety.

Communication : reassure and inform the patient.

Communication plays a crucial role in the patient experience in nuclear medicine. Given that this speciality is less familiar to the general public than other medical fields, and that it involves the use of radioactive substances, patients may feel a degree of apprehension or anxiety. Effective communication is therefore essential to reassure, educate and guide patients through the process.

1. Active listening :
   Understanding concerns: Taking the time to listen to the patient's concerns and questions helps to target the information to be provided.

   Validating emotions: Acknowledging and validating the patient's feelings, whether anxious, curious or otherwise, is the first step in establishing a relationship of trust.

2. Clear and appropriate information :
   Accessible language: Even if the target audience is mainly nurses, it is crucial to express yourself clearly and simply when speaking directly to the patient, avoiding medical jargon wherever possible.

   Visual aids: Using diagrams, brochures or videos can help patients understand the procedure better.

3. Anticipating questions :
   Explain the process: Describe step-by-step what the patient should expect, from preparation to the actual examination and follow-up.

   Risks and benefits: Explain why the examination is necessary, what it may reveal, and what the possible alternatives are. It is also crucial to discuss the associated risks, even if they are minimal.

4. Encourage interaction :
   Ask questions: Encourage patients to ask questions and express their concerns.

   Honest answers: If a question cannot be answered immediately, it's best to admit it and commit to providing an answer as soon as possible.

5. Establish a climate of trust :
   Empathetic attitude: Showing empathy and understanding can greatly reassure the patient.

   Confidentiality: Assuring patients that all information concerning them is treated with the utmost care and confidentiality.

6. Post-review information :

- **What to expect:** Inform the patient about how they may feel after the examination and give them advice to help them recover.
- **Follow-up:** Explain when and how the results will be communicated and what the next steps will be.

Communication is a powerful tool for transforming a potentially stressful experience into a reassuring and educational one for the patient. A well-informed patient is generally more relaxed and cooperative, which makes the examination or treatment go more smoothly.

Chapter 3:
SPECIFIC PROCEDURES AND INTERVENTIONS

The different types of scintigraphy.

Scintigraphy is a medical imaging technique that uses radiopharmaceuticals to visualise and assess the function of different organs or tissues. Based on the detection of radiation emitted by these substances once administered to the patient, it offers a functional rather than anatomical view, unlike techniques such as CT or MRI. Several types of scintigraphy are performed depending on the organ or pathology targeted.

1. Bone scan :
   Objective: To assess bone activity, particularly in cases of unexplained pain, bone metastases or fractures not visible on X-rays.
   Radiopharmaceutical commonly used: technetium-99m.
2. Cardiac scintigraphy :
   Objective: to examine blood flow in the heart muscle and assess areas of infarction or ischaemia.
   Radiopharmaceutical commonly used: Thallium-201 or Technetium-99m.
3. Thyroid scan :
   Objective: To assess the function and morphology of the thyroid gland and detect nodules or inflammation.
   Radiopharmaceutical commonly used: Iodine-123 or Technetium-99m.
4. Lung scintigraphy :
   Objective: To detect pulmonary embolism and assess ventilation and pulmonary perfusion.

Radiopharmaceutical commonly used: Technetium-99m.

5. Renal scintigraphy :

Objective: To assess the function and structure of the kidneys and detect obstructions or inflammation.

Radiopharmaceutical commonly used: Technetium-99m.

6. Hepatobiliary scintigraphy :

Objective: To study the function of the liver and bile ducts and detect obstructions or inflammation.

Radiopharmaceutical commonly used: iminodiacetic labelled technetium-99m.

7. Parathyroid scintigraphy :

Objective: To locate the hyperactive parathyroid glands in cases of hyperparathyroidism.

Radiopharmaceutical commonly used: Technetium-99m or Sestamibi.

8. Scintigraphy of the digestive tract :

Objective: To look for internal bleeding, study motility or identify inflammations such as Crohn's disease.

Radiopharmaceutical commonly used: Technetium-99m.

Each of these scans provides valuable insight into the function and condition of the organ being studied, helping to diagnose, plan treatment and monitor pathologies. Before a scan is carried out, specific preparation may be required, and it is essential to inform and reassure the patient about the safety and conduct of the examination.

Radionuclide therapies.

Radionuclide therapies, also known as radioisotope therapies, represent a unique approach to the treatment of various pathologies, mainly oncological. Instead of using only external radiation to treat a disease (as in external radiotherapy), radionuclide therapies use radioactive isotopes administered to the patient to specifically target certain cells or tissues.

1. Basic principle :

Radioactive isotopes are either ingested, injected or implanted directly into the body. These isotopes emit radiation that can destroy diseased cells while sparing the surrounding healthy tissue to a large extent.

2. Types of radionuclide therapy :

Radioimmunotherapy :

Uses antibodies labelled with radioisotopes to specifically target tumour cells.

Example: Treatment of non-Hodgkin's lymphoma with ibritumomab tiuxetan (Zevalin).

Radiolabelled peptide therapy :

Peptides, which bind to receptors on tumour cells, are labelled with radioactive isotopes.

Example: Treatment of neuroendocrine tumours with DOTATATE labelled with Lutetium-177.

Radionuclide therapy for the thyroid :

Uses radioactive iodine (I-131) to treat thyroid disorders, whether cancer or hyperthyroidism.

Radioembolization :

Radiolabelled microspheres are introduced into the arteries supplying a tumour, usually in the liver, to deliver radiation locally and obstruct the blood supply to the tumour.

Example: Yttrium-90 radioembolisation for liver tumours.

Radium-223 dichloride :

Used to treat bone metastases from castration-resistant prostate cancer.

3. Advantages :

Precise targeting: Radionuclides can be designed to specifically target diseased cells, thereby reducing side effects.

Systemic treatment: These can treat metastases throughout the body, not just a localised tumour.
4. Precautions and side effects :
   Like all medical treatments, radionuclide therapies carry risks and side effects. These can vary depending on the type of therapy, the dose administered and the individual.
   Close medical supervision is essential before, during and after treatment to optimise results and manage adverse effects.
5. The future of radionuclide therapies :
   With advances in nuclear research, new radioisotopes and more precise targeting methods are being developed. This could potentially pave the way for more effective and less toxic therapies for various pathologies.

Radionuclide therapies offer a promising treatment option, particularly for patients who do not respond to traditional treatments or who are looking for alternatives to invasive surgery.

The role of the nurse in PET-CT.

Positron Emission Tomography-Computed Tomography (PET-CT) is a highly specialised medical imaging method that combines the advantages of PET and CT to provide both functional and anatomical images. It is mainly used to detect and assess the extent of various pathologies, including many cancers.
The role of the nurse in this area is crucial in several respects:

1. Preparing the patient :
   Preliminary interview: Gather essential information (medical history, allergies, medication taken) and

check the suitability of the PET-CT scan (for example, by ensuring that the patient is not pregnant).

Physical preparation: Make sure the patient is well hydrated, give instructions about fasting beforehand, and sometimes administer sedatives or anxiolytics for anxious patients.

2. Administration of the radiopharmaceutical :

Injection of the radiolabelled tracer, often based on fluorine-18 FDG (fluorodeoxyglucose), into the patient's bloodstream. The nurse must ensure correct and safe administration, while monitoring for possible patient reactions.

3. Patient monitoring :

After the injection, the patient often has to wait a set period of time (usually 45 minutes to 1 hour) before the scan itself. During this time, the nurse monitors the patient's well-being, makes sure they remain calm and answers any questions they may have.

4. Assistance during the examination :

Although the machine is generally operated by a nuclear medicine technologist, the nurse is often present to assist the patient, in particular by helping them to position themselves correctly and reassuring them.

5. Post-examination care :

Provide post-procedure instructions, such as drinking plenty of water to help eliminate the radiopharmaceutical from the body.

Monitor for any post-administration reactions to the tracer and take appropriate action if necessary.

6. Communication and education :

Inform patients about the procedure, answer their questions and reassure them.

Working closely with radiologists and technologists to ensure that the examination runs smoothly.

7. Risk management :
  Knowing and strictly applying safety protocols to minimise radiation exposure for both patients and staff.
8. Administrative and logistical tasks :
  Helping to manage appointments, prepare radiopharmaceutical doses and keep patients' medical records up to date.

The role of the PET/CT nurse is multidimensional, requiring a combination of technical, clinical and interpersonal skills. At the heart of the procedure, the nurse acts as a link between the patient, the technology and the medical team, ensuring that the examination runs safely and efficiently.

Collaboration
with the interdisciplinary team.

In nuclear medicine, as in many other medical fields, interdisciplinary collaboration is essential to ensure that patients receive the best possible overall care. Nurses, often considered to be the central pillar of this care, work in close collaboration with various professionals. This interdisciplinary collaboration plays a crucial role in guaranteeing the quality of care, patient safety and diagnostic accuracy.

1. Radiologists and nuclear medicine physicians :
  These specialists interpret the images and test results. Close collaboration with the nurse ensures that the relevant clinical data are taken into account in the interpretation.
2. Nuclear medicine technologists :
  They operate the machines and carry out the imaging examinations directly. They work with the nurses to

prepare the patient, position the patient correctly and obtain the best possible quality images.

3. Pharmacists, in particular radiopharmacists :

They prepare and supply the radiopharmaceuticals needed for the examinations. Regular communication with the nurses is essential to ensure that the right doses are administered at the right time.

4. Oncologists and other medical specialists :

These doctors refer their patients for nuclear medicine examinations. The nurse often plays the role of coordinator, ensuring that all relevant information is shared and that the patient is well prepared for the examination.

5. Medical physicists :

They ensure that the equipment is working properly and that radiological safety is maintained. The nurse works closely with them to ensure that protocols are followed and that radiation doses are minimised.

6. Social workers and psychologists :

Some patients, particularly those with serious diagnoses such as cancer, may require psychological or social support. Nurses can identify these needs and facilitate contact with these professionals.

7. Other nurses and care assistants :

They often provide direct patient care and may have important clinical information that can influence the performance or interpretation of the examination.

The collaborative nature of nuclear medicine requires nurses not only to be competent in their own speciality, but also to have excellent communication and teamwork skills. The ultimate aim of this interdisciplinary collaboration is to ensure comprehensive patient care, from preparation to interpretation and post-examination follow-up.

Chapter 4:
SAFETY IN NUCLEAR MEDICINE

Protection against radiation :
for both patient and professional.

Nuclear medicine, by its very nature, involves the use of radioactive substances. These materials, although beneficial in the diagnosis and treatment of various medical conditions, require strict precautions to protect both patients and professionals from the potentially harmful effects of radiation.

Patient protection :
1. ALARA (As Low As Reasonably Achievable) principle :
 Justification: Ensure that each procedure is medically justified.
 Optimisation: Use the minimum dose necessary to obtain the required diagnostic information.
 Limitation: Ensure that the dose received by an individual does not exceed the limits recommended for the general public.
2. Education and information :
 Explain the procedure clearly to the patient, including the benefits and risks.
 Advise the patient on post-procedure measures, such as the importance of drinking plenty of water to help eliminate the radiopharmaceuticals quickly.
3. Careful selection of radiopharmaceuticals :
 Use agents that are rapidly eliminated from the body and present a low risk of residual radiation.
Protection of professionals :
1. PPE (Personal Protective Equipment) :
 Use lead aprons, protective shields, gloves and other accessories to minimise direct exposure.

2. Dosimeters :
   Wear dosimeters to continuously monitor radiation exposure.
3. Regular training :
   Providing ongoing training in radiological safety to keep abreast of best practice and the latest research.
4. Use of specialised tools :
   Use tongs and shields to handle radioactive sources and avoid direct exposure.
5. Installation design :
   Specially designed rooms with leaded walls to minimise radiation dispersion.
   Appropriate storage areas for radioactive waste.
6. Working protocols :
   Establish work routines that minimise the time spent near radioactive sources and maximise the distance between the professional and the source.
7. Waste management :
   Follow strict procedures for the management, storage and disposal of radioactive waste.

It is essential to stress that nuclear medicine procedures, when carried out correctly and following safety protocols, are safe for patients and professionals alike. However, vigilance, ongoing training and strict compliance with guidelines are essential to guarantee this safety.

Radioactive waste management.

Managing radioactive waste is a crucial part of nuclear medicine. This waste arises from the use of radiopharmaceuticals and other radioactive materials used for diagnostic and therapeutic purposes. Appropriate management of this waste is essential to protect patients, healthcare professionals and the environment from the potentially harmful effects of radiation.

1. Classification of radioactive waste :
Waste is generally classified according to its level of radioactivity and its radioactive lifetime:

Very low-level waste: items that have been in contact with radioactive materials but have low radioactivity.

Low- and intermediate-level waste: For example, syringes, vials and other materials used to administer radiopharmaceuticals.

High-level waste: Less common in nuclear medicine, this waste generally comes from industries such as nuclear power plants.

2. Storage and containment :

Temporary storage: Waste is often stored on site for a period of time to allow radioactivity to decrease. Leaded containers can be used to minimise the dispersion of radiation.

Long-term storage: In facilities specially designed to manage radioactivity over long periods.

3. Waste treatment :

Compaction: Reducing the volume of waste by compacting it.

Incineration: Some waste can be incinerated following strict protocols to reduce volume and eliminate organic components.

Solidification: Encapsulating waste in a solid material, such as cement, to stabilise it.

4. Disposal :

Surface disposal: Low-level waste is often buried in specific sites designed to contain radioactivity.

Deep disposal: Higher-level waste can be stored deep underground in geological facilities.

5. Monitoring and control :

All waste and storage areas must be regularly monitored to detect any leaks or other problems.

Storage facilities must be checked regularly to ensure their integrity.

6. Training and education :
   It is essential that all personnel involved in the handling, treatment and disposal of radioactive waste are properly trained and keep their knowledge up to date.
7. Regulatory and legal liability :
   Each country generally has strict regulations concerning the management of radioactive waste. Healthcare establishments must ensure that they comply with all legal and regulatory requirements.

Effective management of radioactive waste in nuclear medicine requires careful planning, appropriate training, regular monitoring and constant accountability. This is essential to protect public health and the environment.

Emergency situations and response to incidents.

Emergency situations in nuclear medicine can range from minor incidents, such as a small spill of radioactive material, to more serious events, such as significant exposure to radiation. In all cases, preparation, rapid reaction and knowledge of protocols are essential to ensure safety.

1. Emergency preparedness :
   Training: All professionals working in nuclear medicine must be trained to respond to emergency situations. This includes knowledge of emergency protocols, handling of radioactive material and basic first aid.
   Equipment: Have the necessary tools at hand, such as spill kits, Geiger counters, protective clothing and specific antidotes.

2. Common scenarios :

Spillage of radioactive materials: In the event of a spill, immediately isolate the area, wear appropriate PPE, clean up the spill using absorbent materials and place the waste in a sealed container.

Accidental exposure to radiation: If a professional or patient is accidentally exposed to a high dose of radiation, it is crucial to assess the dose received, consult a radiation protection specialist and, if necessary, administer appropriate treatment.

Accidents when handling equipment: This can include equipment failure or human error leading to unexpected exposures. In such cases, it is crucial to stop the equipment immediately, evacuate the area if necessary and report the incident.

3. Communication :

Immediately inform management and those responsible for radiological safety.

If necessary, alert the appropriate health and safety authorities.

Communicate clearly and calmly with all those involved to ensure a coordinated response.

4. Post-incident assessment :

Once the situation has been brought under control, it is crucial to carry out a full assessment to understand what happened, the contributing factors and the measures to be taken to avoid future incidents.

Records must be kept up to date with precise details of the incident, the people involved, the actions taken and recommendations for the future.

5. Review of protocols :

Incidents, even minor ones, should be used as an opportunity to learn and improve safety and training protocols.

6. Psychological support :

Radiological accidents can have an emotional impact on victims, whether patients or healthcare professionals. It is crucial to offer psychological support to those who need it.

The key to effectively managing emergency situations in nuclear medicine is thorough preparation, regular training, effective communication and continuous review of protocols and procedures to ensure everyone's safety.

Chapter 5:
ETHICS AND PROFESSIONALISM

Informed consent in nuclear medicine.

Informed consent is a fundamental pillar of ethical medical practice, guaranteeing the patient's right to be informed and to make informed decisions about their own body and health. In nuclear medicine, given the implications associated with exposure to radiation and the use of radioactive substances, informed consent is of particular importance.

1. The principles of informed consent :
    Autonomy: Every patient has the right to make decisions about his or her own body.
    Beneficence: The action taken must be in the patient's best interest.
    Non-maleficence: Not causing harm to the patient.
    Justice: Patients must be treated fairly and equally.
2. Informing the patient :
    Nature of the examination: The patient must clearly understand what the examination is, how it is carried out and why it is necessary.
    Associated risks: All possible risks, however minimal, must be clearly communicated. This includes side effects of radiopharmaceuticals, risks associated with radiation exposure, etc.
    Benefits: The potential benefits of the procedure should be explained, including how it may aid diagnosis or treatment.
    Alternatives: If other methods of diagnosis or treatment exist, they should be presented.

3. The consent process :

Open discussion: It is essential to give patients the opportunity to ask questions and discuss their concerns.

Documentation: Once the patient has given consent, this must be documented. A written consent form is usually signed by the patient and the healthcare professional.

Withdrawal: It is crucial to inform patients that they have the right to withdraw their consent at any time, without any detriment to their care.

4. Consent for special populations :

Children: In most jurisdictions, a parent or guardian must give consent for medical procedures performed on minors.

Patients unable to give consent: For patients with intellectual disabilities, suffering from mental disorders or unable to understand information, consent must be obtained through a legal guardian or a legal representative.

5. Challenges in nuclear medicine :

Complexity of procedures: Nuclear medicine procedures can be technical and difficult for ordinary people to understand. It is therefore essential to explain things simply and clearly.

Associated risks: The idea of radiation can cause anxiety. The professional must approach this subject delicately, reassuring the patient while providing accurate information.

Informed consent in nuclear medicine is not simply a matter of obtaining a signature on a form. It is an interactive process that requires communication, listening and respect.

Professional secrecy and confidentiality.

Professional secrecy and confidentiality are fundamental principles of medical practice. They guarantee the protection of patient privacy and reinforce the trust between patients and healthcare professionals. In nuclear medicine, as in all areas of medicine, these principles are essential to ensure ethical and professional care.

1. Definition and importance :

Professional secrecy: Obligation on healthcare professionals not to divulge information entrusted to them by a patient.

Confidentiality: Protecting a patient's medical, personal and other information from unauthorised disclosure.

2. Why is this essential?

Trust: Patients are more inclined to share information relevant to their care if they know it will remain confidential.

Dignity and respect: Every patient has the right to privacy.

Ethical and professional standards: Respect for professional secrecy is an ethical obligation.

3. Implementation in nuclear medicine :

Medical records: These must be stored securely, with access restricted to authorised professionals only.

Clinical discussions: All conversations concerning a patient must take place away from prying ears.

Use of technology: When sending images or data electronically, it is crucial to use secure and encrypted systems.

4. Limits of professional secrecy :
Although essential, professional secrecy is not absolute. In certain circumstances, it can be broken, in particular :

Patient consent: If the patient agrees to share information.

Legal obligation: In certain cases, the law may require the disclosure of information, for example in the case of notifiable diseases.

Imminent risk: If the patient represents a threat to themselves or others.

5. Ethical dilemmas :
There may be times when healthcare professionals find themselves faced with dilemmas concerning confidentiality, particularly when they feel that it would be in the patient's best interests to share information, but that this would run counter to professional secrecy.

6. Training and awareness :
It is essential that all healthcare professionals, including those working in nuclear medicine, receive appropriate training on the importance of professional secrecy and best practices for ensuring confidentiality.

Professional secrecy and confidentiality are pillars of ethical medical practice. They protect patient privacy, strengthen the patient-professional relationship and guarantee respectful and dignified care.

Continuing education :
Keeping up to date in an evolving field.

Nuclear medicine is a highly specialised, dynamic and constantly evolving field, with regular technological advances, new research and changes in clinical practice. For nurses and other healthcare professionals working in this sector, continuing education is therefore not only beneficial, but often essential to ensuring the quality of patient care.

1. Why is continuing education crucial?

Evolving technologies: With the emergence of new equipment and software, it's essential to keep up to date and be trained in their optimal use.

Updating knowledge: Medical research is advancing at a rapid pace. New studies can change our understanding of a disease or the best treatment practices.

Standards and regulations: Clinical guidelines, government regulations and professional association recommendations are subject to change, requiring regular updating.

Improving skills: Ongoing training helps to refine and develop skills, ensuring optimum patient care.

2. Continuing education :

Workshops and seminars: These meetings enable professionals to learn directly from recognised experts in the field.

Conferences and congresses: These events bring together numerous experts and offer training sessions, demonstrations and presentations of recent research.

Online training: Thanks to technology, many continuing education programmes are available online, enabling flexible learning.

Internships and residencies: Some professionals may choose to spend time in another establishment to acquire specific skills.

3. Importance of certification :

Professional recognition: Certification can attest to an individual's skills in a specialist area of nuclear medicine.

Quality assurance: This guarantees employers, colleagues and patients that the professional has a certain level of competence.

Career opportunities: Certification can open the door to more advanced or specialist positions.

4. Challenges and obstacles :

Time: Finding time in a busy schedule to take a course can be difficult.

Costs: Further training can be expensive, although some employers may offer financial assistance or grants.

Relevance: Not all courses are created equal. It is essential to choose programmes that are relevant and recognised.

5. Personal liability :

Although employers and professional associations play a role in promoting continuing education, it is ultimately up to individual professionals to take responsibility for their own development and invest in their own continuing education.

In the constantly changing landscape of nuclear medicine, continuing education is an invaluable tool for ensuring high-quality care, remaining competent and developing professionally. It not only enhances individual skills, but also elevates the profession as a whole.

Chapter 6:
TESTIMONIALS AND CLINICAL CASES

Nurses dealing with rare cases.

Nuclear medicine, with its unique approach to diagnosis and treatment, can sometimes bring nurses into contact with rare or atypical cases. These situations can be stimulating, but also a source of anxiety, as they are outside the normal routine and require special attention.

1. Recognise the uniqueness of each case:
Every patient is unique, and although the majority of cases follow a familiar pattern, there will always be exceptions. These cases may arise from a rare disease, an atypical response to treatment or an unusual clinical presentation.

2. The importance of training and experience :
While solid basic training is essential, it is experience that best prepares nurses to deal with the unexpected. By encountering a variety of cases and learning from each situation, nurses accumulate a wealth of knowledge that will help them in future situations.

3. Team support :
When faced with a rare case, it is essential to draw on the collective expertise of the medical team. Working with radiopharmacists, nuclear physicians, technologists and other nurses can offer new perspectives and innovative solutions.

4. Research and resources :
Nurses may need to consult medical literature, take part in specialist forums or contact experts in the field to obtain further information on a rare case.

5. Communication with the patient :
Patients themselves may feel anxious or uncertain when faced with a rare situation. Nurses play a key role in informing and reassuring patients and answering their

questions. It is important to provide accurate information, while avoiding medical jargon.

6. Managing uncertainty :
Faced with a rare case, nurses may feel uncertain. This is normal. It's essential to acknowledge these feelings, accept that it's impossible to know everything and actively seek solutions.

7. Documentation :
Meticulous documentation of the care provided, observations and reactions of the patient is crucial. These notes can be a valuable reference for future treatment of the patient and other similar cases.

8. Sharing knowledge :
After managing a rare case, it can be beneficial to share this experience with colleagues at team meetings or professional conferences. This can help other professionals prepare for similar situations.

9. Personal well-being :
Rare cases can be stressful. Nurses must take care of themselves, seeking support if necessary and practising relaxation or stress management techniques.

Although rare cases in nuclear medicine can present challenges, they also offer an opportunity for learning and professional growth. They remind nurses of the importance of remaining curious, continually striving to improve their skills and valuing the support of their colleagues and the medical community.

Managing emotions : the ups and downs of the job.

The role of the nurse in nuclear medicine, as in many other areas of healthcare, is emotionally charged. In addition to their technical and clinical responsibilities, nurses are often the first to interact with patients, supporting them in their concerns and sharing their moments of relief or disappointment. This emotional closeness can have a profound impact on nurses' well-being. Addressing this reality with sensitivity is essential to preserving the mental and emotional health of the professional while providing exceptional patient care.

1. Rewarding moments :

Successful diagnoses: When a patient receives reassuring news following an examination, the satisfaction they feel is immense.

Building relationships: The trust and bonds forged with patients and their families are intangible rewards of the profession.

Contributing to medical science: Participating in the advancement of nuclear medicine and improving treatments is a source of pride.

2. Difficult times :

Bad news: Telling a patient about a serious illness or an unfavourable outcome can be heartbreaking.

Complex situations: Some cases can be both medically and emotionally complicated.

Constant stress: The hectic pace, the need to deal with emergencies and the weight of responsibilities can be exhausting.

3. Strategies for managing emotions :

Peer supervision and support: Regular discussions with colleagues allow you to share experiences, get advice and feel supported.

Stress management training: These courses can provide practical tools for dealing with the emotional demands of the job.

Mindfulness and meditation: These practices help you to stay centred and manage your emotions with serenity.

4. The importance of disconnection :
    Regular breaks: Taking the time to relax, even briefly, helps you recharge your batteries.
    Holidays: Getting away from work to rest and enjoy yourself is essential for preventing burnout.
5. Recognising the signs of burnout :
    Physical symptoms: Chronic fatigue, headaches, sleep disorders.
    Emotional symptoms: Irritability, sadness, anxiety or disinterest in work.
    Behaviours: Isolation, avoidance of tasks or excessive use of alcohol or drugs.
6. Seeking help :
If a nurse is experiencing persistent distress, it is crucial to consult a mental health professional, such as a psychologist or therapist.

The job of a nuclear medicine nurse is undeniably demanding, both technically and emotionally. However, with the right strategies and support, it is possible to navigate through the ups and downs with resilience, compassion and professionalism. The key lies in recognising one's own emotions, seeking support and committing to personal well-being.

The importance of teamwork in nuclear medicine.

Nuclear medicine, with its advanced technology and specific applications, requires close collaboration between different healthcare professionals. Teamwork is not only essential to ensure the safety and effectiveness of procedures, it is also vital to optimise patient care. Let's take a look at why teamwork is so crucial in nuclear medicine and how it positively influences the care pathway.

1. The interdisciplinary nature of nuclear medicine :
Nuclear medicine is at the crossroads of several specialities, including radiology, radiopharmacy, medical technology and internal medicine. Each professional brings specific expertise to the table, and the success of interventions depends on their ability to work in synergy.

2. Safety and precision :
- **Preparation of radiopharmaceuticals:** Radiopharmacists prepare specific agents for each patient. Clear communication with doctors and nurses is essential to ensure the right dose and the right drug.
- **Image interpretation:** Nuclear physicians and radiologists work together to interpret the images obtained, ensuring accurate diagnoses.

3. Comprehensive patient care :
The medical team ensures that the patient is well informed, prepared and monitored throughout the process, from the moment the appointment is made to post-examination follow-up.

4. Responsiveness and adaptability :
In the event of unforeseen situations, such as an allergic reaction or equipment malfunction, the team must work closely together to make rapid decisions and ensure patient safety.

5. Continuing education and training :
The field of nuclear medicine is constantly evolving. Professionals regularly share their knowledge at training courses, conferences and workshops, reinforcing collective expertise.

6. Emotional support :
Patients visiting nuclear medicine may be anxious or worried. The team works together to provide emotional support, reassure patients and answer their questions.

7. Continuous review and improvement :
The teams frequently carry out case reviews, audits and discussions to assess the processes in place and identify potential improvements.

8. Encourage open communication :
An environment where each member feels free to express their opinions, ask questions or seek help is essential to ensure optimal care.

9. Building confidence :
Mutual trust strengthens team cohesion, enabling each member to rely on the expertise and judgement of his or her colleagues.

Teamwork in nuclear medicine is a cornerstone for ensuring not only the quality of care but also the overall patient experience. Each professional plays a unique role, and it is their collaboration that ensures the smooth running of procedures, patient safety and the quality of diagnosis and treatment.

Chapter 7:
FUNDAMENTALS RADIOBIOLOGY

Understanding biological effects radiation.

Radiation has been both blessed and cursed for its effects on biological tissues. It is used to treat cancer and to diagnose various diseases, but misuse or overexposure can lead to undesirable effects. To understand the biological effects of radiation, it is essential to delve into how radiation interacts with cells and molecules.

1. Initial interaction with matter :
Ionising radiation, such as X-rays and alpha, beta and gamma particles, have the ability to strip electrons from atoms as they pass through matter, creating ions. These ions can disrupt normal molecular functions and cause damage.
2. Direct and indirect damage :
   Direct damage: Radiation can interact directly with molecules, particularly DNA, causing single or double strand breaks.
   Indirect damage: Radiation can ionise water molecules, producing free radicals. These radicals can then react with neighbouring molecules, including DNA, causing damage.

3. Cellular effects :
   Repair: Cells have DNA repair mechanisms that can correct some of the damage caused by radiation.
   Apoptosis: If the damage is too severe, the cell may undergo programmed death to prevent the genetic error from spreading.

Malignant transformation: If a cell damaged by radiation does not die and repair itself properly, it can become malignant, eventually leading to the formation of tumours.

4. Somatic and genetic effects :

Somatic effects: These are effects that manifest themselves in the individual exposed to radiation. This includes acute effects such as radiation sickness, as well as long-term effects such as the development of cancer.

Genetic effects: These effects are observed in the offspring of exposed individuals. They result from damage to germ cells (sperm and egg cells).

5. Factors influencing sensitivity :

Type of radiation: For example, alpha particles are more ionising than gamma rays.

Dose rate: A high dose of radiation received over a short period of time can be more damaging than a low dose spread over a long period.

Type of tissue: Some tissues, such as those that divide rapidly (e.g. bone marrow), are more sensitive to radiation.

6. Thresholds and doses :

It is important to understand that not all the biological effects of radiation have a defined threshold. Some effects, such as carcinogenesis, can occur even at very low doses, although the risk is proportionately low.

7. Protection and prevention :

Knowledge of the biological effects of radiation has led to the development of strict guidelines to protect both patients and healthcare professionals from potential dangers.

Radiation interacts with biological tissues in complex ways. Although we have benefited from radiation in many medical fields, a thorough understanding of its biological effects is essential to minimise the risks and maximise the benefits. Judicious use, combined with adequate protection, ensures that radiation continues to serve humanity safely and effectively.

Interaction mechanisms between radiation and tissue.

The mechanisms of interaction between radiation and tissues are fundamental to understanding the biological effects of radiation. These interactions are at the heart of radiobiology, a field that studies how radiation affects living organisms. Here is a detailed exploration of these mechanisms.

1. Interaction of radiation with atoms :
When radiation passes through matter, it can interact with atoms by knocking off one or more electrons, producing ions. This is why it is called ionising radiation.

2. Production of free radicals :
   Water ionisation: Water makes up around 70% of cell content. When ionised, it can produce highly reactive hydroxyl radicals.
   Chain reactions: These radicals can initiate chain reactions, damaging other molecules in the vicinity.

3. Direct damage to DNA :
Radiation can interact directly with DNA, causing single or double strand breaks, or altering the bases.

4. Indirect damage to DNA :
The free radicals produced by ionisation can react with DNA, also causing breaks or modifications.

5. Types of interaction as a function of radiation :

Photons (X-rays and gamma rays): They can interact by the photoelectric effect, Compton scattering or pair production. The photoelectric effect is dominant at low energies, where a photon is completely absorbed by an atom, releasing an electron. Compton scattering occurs at intermediate energies and involves the deflection of an incident photon with the ejection of an electron. Pair production occurs at very high energies where a photon can be converted into an electron-positron pair near the nucleus.

Alpha particles: These heavy, charged particles have a high ionisation capacity but low penetration. They can cause serious damage over a short distance.

Beta particles: These are electrons or positrons emitted by a nucleus. They penetrate deeper than alpha particles, but cause fewer ionisations per unit distance.

6. Effects of dose and dose rate :

Absorbed dose: This is the energy absorbed per unit mass, measured in gray (Gy).

Dose rate: This is the dose absorbed per unit of time. Radiation with a high dose rate can cause more damage than the same dose administered over a longer period.

7. Tissue sensitivity :

Not all tissues are equally sensitive to radiation. Tissues that are rapidly renewed, such as the skin, bone marrow and intestinal lining, are generally more sensitive.

8. Compensation for damage :

Cells have mechanisms for repairing damaged DNA. However, repair can be imperfect, leading to mutations or cell death.

Understanding the mechanisms of interaction between radiation and tissues is essential for assessing and managing the risks associated with exposure to radiation, whether in a medical, industrial or environmental context.

Stochastic effects vs. deterministic effects.

The effects of ionising radiation on biological tissues can be classified into two main categories: stochastic effects and deterministic effects. Distinguishing between these two types of effects is essential for assessing and managing the risks associated with exposure to radiation.

Stochastic effects :
- **Probabilistic nature:** Stochastic effects have no dose threshold below which the risk is zero. The higher the dose, the greater the risk of a stochastic effect. However, there is no guarantee that an effect will occur, whatever the dose.
- **Independence of severity:** Unlike deterministic effects, the severity of a stochastic effect does not increase with dose. For example, if radiation causes cancer, the severity of the cancer does not depend on the dose received.
- **Examples:** Radiation-induced cancers and genetic mutations are examples of stochastic effects.

Deterministic effects :
- **Dose threshold:** Unlike stochastic effects, deterministic effects generally have a dose threshold below which they do not occur. Once this threshold is reached or exceeded, the effect appears with certainty.
- **Dose-dependent severity:** The severity of the effect increases with the dose of radiation. A low dose may

cause only slight damage, while a high dose may cause severe damage or death.

Examples: Radiation burns, radiation-induced cataracts and acute radiation sickness (symptoms including nausea, vomiting, diarrhoea and hair loss) are examples of deterministic effects.

Some key points to remember:

Radiological protection: In radiological protection, the principles of dose limitation have been established primarily to reduce the risk of stochastic effects. For this reason, permissible doses for exposed workers and the general public are set at levels well below the thresholds for deterministic effects.

Dose and response: For stochastic effects, the dose-response relationship is generally considered to be linear with no threshold. This means that even a small dose can theoretically increase the risk. For deterministic effects, once the threshold is exceeded, the risk increases rapidly with increasing dose.

The distinction between stochastic and deterministic effects is fundamental to understanding the risks associated with radiation and to establishing appropriate radiation protection standards. Each type of effect presents unique health and safety concerns, and a thorough understanding of both is essential for effective radiological risk management.

Chapter 8:
PSYCHOSOCIAL ASPECTS
IN NUCLEAR MEDICINE

The perception of radioactivity
and the associated fears.

Radioactivity, although naturally present in our environment and used in various fields such as medicine, research and energy production, is often shrouded in an aura of mystery and fear. This perception, built up over time, is the result of a combination of ignorance, historical misadventures and often exaggerated representations in the media and popular culture.

Let's take a moment to delve into the complexity of this perception. Ever since the discovery of radioactivity at the end of the 19th century by Henri Becquerel, followed by the work of Marie and Pierre Curie, humanity has been fascinated by this invisible phenomenon that has the power to penetrate matter, illuminate objects in the dark, and treat or even cause disease. The first medical and industrial applications of radioactivity were hailed as miracles of modern science.

However, with the power of this discovery came risks, sometimes underestimated or unknown. The first researchers and workers handling radioactive materials, unaware of the associated dangers, often suffered serious or fatal illnesses. The image of radioactivity has been further tarnished by the major nuclear disasters of the 20th century, such as Chernobyl and Fukushima, which have engraved in the public mind the association between radioactivity and disaster.

The media, in search of captivating stories, have often magnified the dangers of radioactivity, sometimes without context or proportion. Films and novels have depicted mutant monsters and desolate lands, feeding the collective imagination of an invisible and malevolent force. This narrative has reinforced a deep-seated fear of radioactivity, making it a taboo subject that is poorly understood by the general public.

This fear is heightened by the impalpable nature of radioactivity. Undetectable by our senses, it embodies the unknown, and as the writer H.P. Lovecraft said, "The oldest and strongest emotion of mankind is fear, and the oldest and strongest of fears is the fear of the unknown."

However, despite this fear, it is essential to understand radioactivity in all its complexity, recognising its dangers while accepting its many benefits. In a world where science plays an increasingly important role, a balanced understanding of radioactivity, based on facts and not myths, is crucial if we are to tackle the challenges of our time with serenity and fully exploit the potential of this mysterious and powerful energy.

Supporting the patient : managing anxiety and expectations.

In the world of nuclear medicine, as in other medical fields, patient support is fundamental. The potentially invasive nature of the procedures, combined with the unknown nature of radioactivity, can generate feelings of anxiety and worry in patients. As a result, the nurse's ability to manage this anxiety and meet the patient's expectations is essential to ensure an optimal and humane experience.

Anxiety about a medical examination, whether diagnostic or therapeutic, is a normal reaction. The thought of facing the unknown, combined with the fear of the results, can be a source of deep unease. Add to this the word 'radioactivity', often charged with negative images in the collective imagination, and you have a potential recipe for a stressful experience.

The nurse plays a central role in reassuring and preparing the patient. Open and transparent communication is crucial. The simple act of explaining how the examination will be carried out, why it is being done and what it will involve, can dispel many fears. Humans tend to fear what they don't understand, so by shedding light on the mystery, the nurse reduces the unknown that causes anxiety.

But beyond simple communication, it's all about empathy and listening. Every patient is unique, with his or her own concerns and needs. Some want detailed explanations, while others prefer a more reassuring approach. Nurses need to be aware of these differences and adapt their approach accordingly.

The patient's expectations are just as important. Some hope for immediate results, while others may have concerns about side effects or the long-term implications of the examination. Clarifying what the patient can expect from the examination, and what they should not, is fundamental to avoiding disappointment or unnecessary worry.

Finally, the importance of a warm and welcoming environment should not be underestimated. From the waiting room to the examination room, creating a soothing environment can make a big difference to a patient's perception. Soft music, soothing decor or even a simple warm blanket can transform a cold clinical experience into a much more human one.

The role of the nurse in nuclear medicine, or in any other medical field, goes far beyond the purely technical. It is a role of accompaniment, education and support. By putting the patient at the heart of the process, by listening and responding to their needs and concerns, nurses contribute not only to a better patient experience but also to better clinical outcomes. Comprehensive care, in which the patient feels heard, understood and supported, is the key to truly people-centred medicine.

Working with psychologists or social workers.

Nuclear medicine, like other medical specialities, does not operate in silos. It is part of a medical ecosystem in which different professionals work together to provide holistic patient care. Among these professionals, psychologists and social workers play a crucial role. Their collaboration with nuclear medicine nurses is essential to address the emotional, psychosocial and sometimes economic aspects associated with care.

When faced with an illness, invasive examinations or therapy, patients can experience a whole range of emotions: anxiety, depression, fear, uncertainty, anger, even denial. While nurses are trained to deal with some of these emotions, it is sometimes necessary to call on a specialist professional for more in-depth care. This is where the psychologist comes in. He or she offers a place to listen and talk, enabling patients to express their emotions, understand them and learn how to manage them.

Social workers, for their part, intervene to support the patient as a whole, particularly in terms of social support. They can help patients navigate the administrative maze of the healthcare system, find solutions to financial problems or mobilise resources for care at home. In addition, in the event of serious illness, social workers can provide support for the patient's family, suggest suitable accommodation or transport solutions, or refer them to associations or support groups.

Collaboration between the nurse, psychologist and social worker is therefore essential to provide comprehensive care. This collaboration involves regular communication between these professionals. They share relevant information (while respecting professional confidentiality), refer patients to each other according to identified needs, and draw up coordinated care plans.

Nuclear medicine nurses must therefore be able to recognise the signs of psychological distress or social difficulties in their patients and know when and how to refer them to the right professional. Similarly, they must be prepared to receive information and advice from psychologists and social workers to provide better support for patients.

Treatment in nuclear medicine, as in other medical fields, is a team effort. Each professional makes his or her own contribution, and it is this interdisciplinary collaboration that enables us to offer patients comprehensive care that respects their medical, psychological and social needs.

Chapter 9:
WORKING TOGETHER
WITH OTHER MEDICAL SERVICES

Liaison with oncology : a key partnership.

Nuclear medicine and oncology are two closely related medical disciplines, and their interaction is essential for optimal care of cancer patients. Indeed, their collaboration is often synonymous with accurate diagnosis, personalised treatment and rigorous follow-up, offering patients the best chance of recovery or management of their disease.

Nuclear medicine provides oncology with a range of invaluable diagnostic and therapeutic tools. For example, Positron Emission Tomography (PET) is regularly used to detect, localise and assess the progression of tumours. This type of imaging not only shows the location and size of the tumour, but also its metabolic activity, providing a dynamic view of the disease.

Nuclear medicine also offers radionuclide therapies, using radioactive isotopes to target and destroy specific cancer cells. This therapeutic approach is sometimes an alternative or a complement to more conventional treatments such as surgery, chemotherapy or radiotherapy.

However, collaboration between nuclear medicine and oncology is not just limited to the technical aspect. It is above all a human synergy, where oncologists and nuclear medicine specialists regularly discuss patients' cases. They discuss imaging results, evaluate treatment options together, and coordinate their interventions to ensure smooth, coherent care.

The interaction between these two specialities is also essential for patient follow-up. While the oncologist monitors the clinical course and any side-effects of treatment, the nuclear medicine specialist can provide valuable insights into the course of the disease at a molecular or cellular level. Together, they work to adjust current treatments if necessary and anticipate the next steps.

What's more, this collaboration is enriching from an academic and research point of view. By working hand in hand, the two disciplines can push back the frontiers of knowledge, develop new diagnostic and therapeutic methods and continually improve the care of cancer patients.

The link between nuclear medicine and oncology is much more than just a technical collaboration. It is a key partnership, based on trust, communication and the sharing of expertise, which aims to offer patients comprehensive, integrated and above all humane care. In the fight against cancer, this multidisciplinary synergy is a major asset, putting technology and people at the service of healing.

Working in tandem with radiology.

Nuclear medicine and radiology, although two distinct disciplines, often work in tandem to provide a complete and accurate picture of a patient's health. Their alliance is crucial to maximising the diagnostic and therapeutic benefits for patients.

At its core, radiology uses radiation (such as X-rays) to create detailed images of the anatomical structures of the body. Modalities such as radiography, computed tomography (CT) and magnetic resonance imaging (MRI) provide precise images of bones, organs and other body structures.

On the other hand, nuclear medicine uses small quantities of radioactive material to diagnose, assess and treat disease. It provides functional images, showing how organs function, rather than just how they look.

When these two disciplines are combined, as in the case of PET-CT, they allow a fusion of precise anatomy with function, offering a complete perspective of health and disease. CT provides the detailed anatomical image while PET reveals the metabolic activity, allowing areas of abnormal metabolic concern to be precisely located within the anatomical context.

Working in tandem with radiology offers a number of advantages:

Greater diagnostic accuracy: Combining the strengths of the two modalities can help to detect, locate and characterise diseases with greater precision.

Targeted treatment: Nuclear medicine can use the anatomical information provided by radiology to precisely target radionuclide treatments.

Optimised monitoring: The ability to monitor both anatomy and function can help doctors assess the effectiveness of treatments and adjust therapeutic approaches as required.

Research and development: Together, these disciplines can carry out advanced studies, developing new imaging or therapeutic techniques.

Collaboration is not just about machines and technologies. It also extends to the medical teams. Radiologists and nuclear medicine specialists hold regular joint meetings, sharing their expertise to discuss complex cases, exchange perspectives and ensure optimum patient care.

Nuclear medicine and radiology working in tandem illustrates the importance of interdisciplinary collaboration in medicine. Each brings its own strengths to the table, and their alliance makes it possible to optimise patient care, offering accurate diagnoses, effective treatments and, ultimately, medical care of the highest quality.

Relations with the surgery department and other specialities.

The nuclear medicine department plays a cross-disciplinary role within the hospital, interacting with a multitude of medical specialities. Among these interactions, relations with the surgery department are particularly crucial, but other specialties also rely heavily on the expertise of nuclear medicine to optimise patient care.

Surgery department:
> **Pre-operative location**: Prior to certain surgical procedures, it is essential to precisely locate areas of interest, whether tumours, sentinel lymph nodes or other structures. Nuclear medicine, using targeted scans, can guide the surgeon to these areas.
> **Post-operative evaluation**: After surgery, nuclear medicine can help to evaluate the success of the operation, detect any complications or monitor the recurrence of the disease.

Other specialities :
> **Cardiology**: Cardiac scans are commonly used to assess heart function and detect areas of ischaemia or infarction.

Endocrinology: Thyroid scans can help detect nodules, assess their function and guide treatments such as iodine radiotherapy.

Nephrology: Nuclear medicine is used to assess kidney function and detect obstructions or reflux.

Neurology: PET brain scans, for example, can be used to assess patients suffering from neurodegenerative diseases such as Alzheimer's.

Respirology: Ventilation and perfusion scans can help detect pulmonary embolism or assess lung function.

Rheumatology: Nuclear medicine can help visualise inflammation in joints or other tissues.

Communication and collaboration :

The success of these interactions relies heavily on effective communication. Nuclear medicine teams need to talk regularly with surgeons and other specialists to understand their specific needs, interpret results in a clinical context and collaborate on therapeutic decision-making.

In addition, multidisciplinary meetings, bringing together surgeons, oncologists, radiologists, nuclear medicine specialists and other healthcare professionals, are often organised to discuss complex cases. These sessions enable a rich exchange of expertise, ensuring that every patient benefits from comprehensive and coherent care.

Nuclear medicine does not operate in silos. Its value lies in its ability to work closely with other specialties, offering unique insights that, when combined with other medical knowledge, ensure the best possible care for every patient.

Chapter 10:
CONTEMPORARY ISSUES AND CHALLENGES

Environmental issues linked to radioactivity.

The field of nuclear medicine, while bringing significant advances in diagnosis and treatment, is not without its environmental concerns related to radioactivity. The management of radioactive isotopes and their potential impact on the environment requires a thorough understanding and strict protocols to ensure the safety of both individuals and the environment.

1. Radioactive waste management :
Hospitals and clinics practising nuclear medicine generate radioactive waste, whether in the form of used syringes, empty vials or other medical equipment. This waste has to be stored safely for a set period of time, until its radioactivity reaches a sufficiently low level to enable it to be disposed of safely. This requires specific facilities, suitable containers and regular monitoring.

2. Waste water and disposal :
After certain examinations or treatments, patients excrete radioactive substances. Although these substances generally have a short half-life, it is essential to ensure that wastewater disposal and treatment systems are capable of managing these elements without harming the environment.

3. Atmospheric emissions :
Some nuclear medicine procedures or equipment can generate low-level radioactive gaseous emissions.

Although these emissions are generally minimal and regulated, it is crucial to monitor and control them to avoid any impact on the environment.

4. Transport and logistics :
Radiopharmaceuticals and other radioactive materials used in nuclear medicine often have to be transported over long distances. This requires specially designed vehicles and strict protocols to avoid any incidents during transport.

5. Natural resources :
The extraction and production of certain isotopes can have an impact on the environment, whether through mining or the use of nuclear reactors to produce specific isotopes. It is therefore essential to ensure that these processes are as environmentally responsible as possible.

6. Awareness-raising and training :
Educating health professionals and the general public about environmental issues related to radioactivity is crucial. A better understanding of the risks and safety protocols can significantly reduce the environmental impact.

7. Research and development :
The constant search for new techniques, less radioactive materials and more environmentally-friendly approaches can help to reduce the ecological footprint of nuclear medicine.

Although nuclear medicine offers considerable benefits in terms of patient care, it also imposes a significant environmental responsibility. By complying with strict standards, investing in research and continually raising awareness among professionals and the public, it is possible to minimise environmental impact while benefiting from the advances made by this medical speciality.

Crisis management:
isotope shortages, world events.

Nuclear medicine, while of crucial importance for the detection and treatment of many diseases, is also subject to a series of unique challenges, particularly in terms of crisis management. Isotope shortages and global events can have a significant impact on the availability and distribution of necessary materials. Let's look at how these situations are managed.

Isotope shortages :

    Anticipation and forecasting: Thanks to constant monitoring of stocks and collaboration with suppliers, institutions can anticipate potential shortages and plan accordingly.

    Optimising use: In the event of a shortage, the use of isotopes can be optimised, by giving priority to the most urgent cases or modifying dosages when it is medically safe to do so.

    Looking for alternatives: It is crucial to look for alternatives to the isotopes in short supply. Sometimes, other types of examination or treatment, although less optimal, can be used temporarily.

    International collaboration: Collaboration with other countries can make it possible to obtain isotopes in times of shortage, particularly if there are problems at the main production facilities.

World events :

    Natural disasters: Events such as earthquakes, floods or hurricanes can disrupt the production or distribution of isotopes. Emergency and business continuity plans must be in place to deal with these situations.

    Political events or conflicts: Geopolitical tensions can affect the availability of isotopes, especially if they come from unstable regions. Diversification of supply sources is essential to reduce this risk.

Global health crises: Situations such as the COVID-19 pandemic can disrupt the supply chain and reduce the availability of resources. Procedures need to be adapted to guarantee the safety of patients and staff, while ensuring continuity of care.

Management strategies :

Planning: Having contingency plans in place to manage various crisis scenarios.

Staff training: Ensure that staff are properly trained to respond to unforeseen situations.

Communication: Maintaining transparent communication with staff, patients and the public is crucial. Inform patients of any changes to their care or treatment as a result of the crisis.

Collaboration: Working closely with other institutions, governments and international bodies can help to share resources and knowledge.

Although nuclear medicine faces unique crisis management challenges, effective planning, training and communication can help mitigate the impact of these situations on patient care.

The future of nuclear medicine: technological and ethical challenges.

Nuclear medicine, as a constantly evolving field of medicine, is at the intersection of cutting-edge technology and important ethical issues. Looking to the future, it is clear that the landscape of nuclear medicine will be shaped by technological innovations and the ethical debates that accompany them. Let's look at these challenges in more detail.

Technological challenges :

Innovations in imaging: New imaging techniques and technologies are constantly emerging, promising higher resolution, greater precision and fewer risks for patients. Integrating these innovations into clinical practice will require in-depth training and financial investment.

Personalised therapies: The trend is towards personalised medicine, where treatments are tailored to a patient's specific genetics and biology. Nuclear medicine will have to develop radiopharmaceuticals targeting specific molecular anomalies.

Robotics and automation: With the advent of robotics, many processes, from the preparation of radiopharmaceuticals to certain aspects of procedures, could be automated, increasing efficiency but also raising questions about the human role in the process.

Ethical challenges :

Access to care: As technology advances, so does its cost. How can we ensure that all patients, regardless of their economic situation, have access to the latest nuclear medicine treatments and technologies?

Informed consent: With treatments becoming increasingly complex, ensuring that patients really understand what they are consenting to is becoming a challenge. Medical staff need to be trained to communicate clearly and effectively.

Privacy and data: New imaging technologies can collect an unprecedented amount of patient data. How is this data stored, shared and protected?

Clinical research: New therapies need to be tested, but how can we ensure that these trials are conducted ethically, respecting the rights and safety of participants?

In the face of these challenges, nuclear medicine will need to demonstrate adaptability and foresight. Ongoing training and adaptability of healthcare professionals will be essential to integrate new technologies while keeping patient safety and well-being at the heart of practice. At the same time, an open ethical dialogue is needed to guide the field through uncharted waters, ensuring that technological advances are always used in a way that is in the best interests of patients and society as a whole.

Chapter 11:
THE WORKING ENVIRONMENT IN NUCLEAR MEDICINE

Specific features of the development premises.

The layout of nuclear medicine facilities has a number of specific features that are essential to guarantee both optimum safety and efficient operation. From design to day-to-day use, every detail counts in providing patients with a safe and comfortable environment, while ensuring the protection of professionals. Let's delve into the subtleties of these unique spaces.

1. Zones dedicated to radioactivity :
  Examination and treatment rooms: These areas require leaded or reinforced concrete walls to limit the spread of radiation. The design of these areas must also allow smooth patient flow and minimise the exposure time for patients and staff.
  Radiopharmaceutical laboratories: These areas are designed for the preparation, storage and handling of radiopharmaceuticals. They require ventilated hoods and shielding to protect against radiation.

2. Secure storage :
Specific areas must be set aside for storing radioactive isotopes, radioactive waste and sensitive equipment. These areas must be secure, with limited access, and built with materials that contain radiation.

3. Waiting areas :
Patients who have received radiopharmaceuticals may need to wait for the drugs to distribute throughout their

body before undergoing tests. These waiting areas must be away from non-radioactive areas and ventilated.

4. Provision for efficiency :
Workflow is crucial. The patient pathway, from reception, preparation and examination to discharge, must be logically designed to minimise travel and exposure.

5. Emergency measures :
Emergency showers and evacuation areas must be provided in the event of a radioactive spill or other incident. Radiation detectors must be installed in strategic locations.

6. Patient comfort :
The environment must be reassuring for the patient. Soothing decor, soft lighting and private areas for changing clothes or discussing treatments can greatly enhance the patient's experience.

7. Staff areas :
Cloakrooms, offices and rest rooms must be provided for staff. The design should also include space for ongoing training, meetings and other administrative needs.

8. Technology and connectivity :
With the rapid evolution of medical technologies, spaces need to be designed to accommodate new equipment. In addition, good connectivity for information systems, such as electronic medical records, is crucial.

The design of premises for nuclear medicine is a subtle balance between safety, efficiency, comfort and technology. Every detail counts, and collaboration between architects, engineers and healthcare professionals is essential to create a space that meets the unique needs of this medical discipline.

Technology at the service of safety.

Nuclear medicine, in essence, deals with radioactive substances for the diagnosis and treatment of various diseases. While this technology brings undeniable health benefits, it also presents challenges in terms of safety. This is where modern technology comes in, offering innovative solutions to maximise the protection of patients, medical staff and the environment.

1. Radiation detectors :
Modern, sophisticated radiation detectors enable exposure levels to be monitored in real time. Whether portable or fixed, these devices are essential for ensuring that levels remain within acceptable limits. Portable detectors, for example, can be worn by staff to monitor their individual exposure.

2. Advanced shielding :
Advances in shielding materials have enabled the creation of more effective barriers against radiation, while at the same time being lighter and more flexible. For example, the lead aprons used by medical staff have evolved to offer better protection while being more comfortable to wear.

3. Digital imaging :
Advances in digital imaging have made it possible to reduce the quantity of radioisotopes needed to obtain a clear image, thereby reducing patients' exposure to radiation.

4. Robotics :
Using robots to handle radioactive materials eliminates the need for humans to handle them directly. This considerably reduces the risk of exposure for laboratory staff and technicians.

5. Specialised software :
Dedicated software helps track the trajectory of radioisotopes in the body, enabling doctors to better plan treatments and ensure that the doses administered are optimal for the patient while minimising side effects.

6. Virtual training :
Simulators and virtual reality give medical staff the opportunity to train in handling radioactive substances in a safe environment, without any real risk.

7. Advanced ventilation systems :
In areas where radioactive substances are handled, specific ventilation systems prevent the spread of radioactive particles, ensuring clean, safe air.

8. Waste management :
Modern technology offers solutions for the treatment, storage and disposal of radioactive waste, ensuring that it is contained safely and effectively.

9. Remote monitoring :
With the rise of IoT (Internet of Things) technologies, it is now possible to remotely monitor equipment, rooms and even patients, to ensure that everything is working properly and safely.

As nuclear medicine continues to evolve, technology plays an essential role in ensuring that this evolution takes place safely. Harmonisation of technology and safety protocols ensures that the benefits of nuclear medicine are realised without compromising the safety of patients, medical staff and the community.

Teamwork :
interactions between doctors, technicians, nurses and other professionals.

In nuclear medicine, as in many medical fields, teamwork is crucial to ensuring optimal patient care. Each member of the team plays a specific and complementary role, and the success of interventions often depends on the ability of different professionals to work together effectively.

1. The nuclear medicine physician :
As the patient's first point of contact, the doctor specialising in nuclear medicine makes the diagnosis, decides on the appropriate treatment and supervises the entire process. He or she assesses the images, interprets the results and liaises with the other specialist doctors to ensure that the patient receives comprehensive care.

2. The nuclear medicine technician :
Technicians are responsible for administering radiopharmaceuticals to patients, performing scans and operating sophisticated equipment. They work closely with the doctor to guarantee the quality of the images obtained and ensure that the examination runs smoothly.

3. The nuclear medicine nurse :
The nurse is often the first point of contact with the patient. They prepare the patient for the examination, administer any necessary medication, monitor the patient's condition during the examination and provide post-examination advice. Nurses are also essential for reassuring patients, answering their questions and supporting them throughout the process.

4. The radiopharmacist :
As an expert in radiopharmaceuticals, the radiopharmacist prepares the radioactive substances required for examinations and treatments. They work in collaboration with the doctor and technician to ensure that the right doses are administered.

5. Other professionals :
Other specialists may be called in depending on the case, including radiologists, surgeons, oncologists and cardiologists. Their expertise is essential for comprehensive patient care, particularly for complex cases or associated pathologies.

6. Administrative staff :
Every medical procedure requires logistical organisation. From secretarial duties to appointment management and billing issues, these professionals play a central role in ensuring that the process runs smoothly.

7. Communication and collaboration :
Effective teamwork relies on fluid communication between all those involved. Regular meetings, shared minutes and modern communication tools are essential to ensure that every member of the team is informed and aligned with the common objectives.

8. Further training and exchanges :
Nuclear medicine is a constantly evolving field. Exchanges between professionals, whether at training courses, conferences or internal meetings, are crucial if we are to remain at the cutting edge of technology and practice.

Nuclear medicine is an orchestrated ballet in which each player, through his or her expertise and collaboration with the other members of the team, contributes to optimal patient care. Synergy and cooperation are the key words in guaranteeing the safety, quality and efficiency of care.

Chapter 12:
EMERGENCY MANAGEMENT
IN NUCLEAR MEDICINE

Recognising vital signs at risk.

Nuclear medicine, by its very nature, can present emergency situations. Although most nuclear medicine procedures are planned and carried out in a controlled environment, unforeseen situations can arise, requiring rapid and decisive action.

Recognising vital signs at risk is an essential skill for any healthcare professional, and in nuclear medicine this ability is all the more crucial because of the specific nature of the discipline.

1. Allergic reactions :
Some patients may experience an allergic reaction to the radiopharmaceuticals or other agents administered. Vital signs to watch out for include wheezing, hives, swelling of the face or throat and rapid heartbeat.

2. Dyspnoea :
Sudden shortness of breath after administration of a radiopharmaceutical may indicate an adverse reaction or complication. Rapid measurement of oxygen saturation, respiratory rate and lung sounds are essential.

3. Hypotension :
A sudden drop in blood pressure may signal a vagal reaction or a more serious reaction to a drug. Regular monitoring of blood pressure and the ability to recognise associated symptoms, such as dizziness, are crucial.

4. Tachycardia or bradycardia :
Cardiac irregularities may occur after the administration of certain agents. Continuous monitoring of heart rhythm and ECG can help detect these abnormalities early.

5. Anxiety and agitation :
Although psychological, these symptoms can affect vital signs. An anxious patient may experience an increase in heart rate and respiratory rate. Calming and reassuring the patient is essential, but it is also important to recognise when further medical intervention is required.

6. Neurological symptoms :
Severe headaches, dizziness, blurred vision or signs of stroke should be taken very seriously, especially if they occur after an operation.

7. Complications associated with venipuncture :
Haematomas, excessive pain or signs of infection around the injection site require special attention.

Emergency response :
  Preparation: Regular training in first aid and emergency procedures is crucial for all team members.
  Emergency equipment: Having a well-equipped and easily accessible emergency trolley is vital. It should contain resuscitation equipment, emergency medicines, a defibrillator and other essential equipment.
  Communication: In an emergency, clear and rapid communication with other members of the team and, if necessary, with external emergency services, is essential.
  Post-incident assessment: After every emergency, it is essential to assess the situation, understand what happened and adjust procedures if necessary.

In nuclear medicine, as in any medical environment, the ability to quickly recognise vital signs at risk and to intervene effectively can mean the difference between life and death. Regular training, adequate preparation and effective communication are the key to effectively managing these emergency situations.

Opposing reactions adiopharmaceuticals.

Radiopharmaceuticals are medical compounds containing radionuclides. They are used in nuclear medicine to diagnose and treat certain diseases. However, like any drug or medical procedure, the administration of radiopharmaceuticals can be accompanied by side effects or adverse reactions. Although they are rare, it is imperative for nurses and other healthcare professionals to be aware of these risks and know how to manage them.
Allergic reactions :

Although extremely rare, allergic reactions can occur after administration of a radiopharmaceutical. These reactions can range from a mild skin rash to life-threatening anaphylaxis. Signs to look out for include skin rash, swelling, difficulty breathing, dizziness and increased heart rate. Prompt treatment is essential in these situations.

Injection site reactions :
Pain, redness or swelling may appear at the injection site. In most cases, these symptoms are mild and disappear rapidly. However, treatment may be required if symptoms persist or worsen.

Systemic reactions :
Nausea, vomiting or a metallic taste in the mouth are sometimes experienced by patients after the administration

of certain radiopharmaceuticals. These symptoms are generally mild and short-lived.

Reactions linked to radioactivity :
It is important to note that the radiopharmaceuticals used in nuclear medicine are designed to minimise the risk associated with radioactivity. The doses used are low, and the radionuclide is generally eliminated rapidly from the body. However, it is essential to comply with the principles of radiation protection to protect both patients and staff.

Managing adverse reactions :

Monitoring: After administration of the radiopharmaceutical, it is essential to monitor the patient for any signs of adverse reaction.

Initial management: In the event of an allergic reaction, the administration of antihistamines or corticosteroids may be necessary. In more serious cases, emergency medical intervention may be required.

Communication: It is crucial to inform patients of the possibility of adverse reactions before administering the radiopharmaceutical and to ask them to inform staff immediately if they feel anything abnormal.

Documentation: Any adverse reaction must be carefully documented in the patient's medical record. This is essential for ongoing monitoring of radiopharmaceutical safety.

Although adverse reactions to radiopharmaceuticals are rare, healthcare professionals in nuclear medicine must be prepared to recognise and manage them effectively to ensure patient safety. Communication, monitoring and ongoing training are essential to minimise these risks.

Rapid response procedures.

Rapid response procedures in nuclear medicine are crucial to the safety of patients and staff. Due to the specific nature of this branch of medicine, emergency situations can be unique and require a tailored approach. However, as in any medical discipline, the main objective is to ensure the safety of the patient and stabilise their condition as quickly as possible.

1. Severe allergic reactions :
    Recognition: Skin rash, difficulty breathing, swelling of the face or throat, dizziness.
    Intervention: Stop any administration in progress, place the patient in a safe position, administer adrenaline in the event of anaphylaxis, call an emergency team.
2. Accidental exposure to radiation :
    Recognition: Leak of a radioactive source, spillage of radioactive material.
    Response: Immediate evacuation of the area, signposting of the area, use of personal protective equipment for the personnel involved, measurement of radioactivity, decontamination if necessary.
3. Ingestion or accidental inhalation of radioactive materials :
    Recognition: Any suspected ingestion or inhalation.
    Intervention: Ensuring the patient's vital stability, administering specific treatments to promote elimination, monitoring the patient's radioactivity.
4. Equipment malfunction during a procedure :
    Recognition: Abnormal noises, alarms, unexpected device shutdown.
    Intervention: Stop the procedure, take the patient to safety, check the patient's condition, call the technical team to assess the device.

5. Adverse reaction to a radiopharmaceutical :

Recognition: Pain at the injection site, signs of allergic reaction, nausea.

Intervention: Close monitoring of the patient, symptomatic treatment, accurate documentation of the incident.

6. Cardiac or respiratory events during the examination :

Recognition: Chest pain, shortness of breath, loss of consciousness.

Intervention: Administration of oxygen, cardiopulmonary resuscitation if necessary, call for an emergency team.

7. Psychological or behavioural incidents :

Recognition: Agitation, excessive anxiety, panic.

Intervention: Attempt to calm the patient using appropriate communication techniques, call in a specialist team if necessary, possible use of light sedation with the patient's consent.

Rapid intervention in nuclear medicine requires specific training and preparation. Procedures must be regularly reviewed and updated to take account of new knowledge and technologies. In addition, regular incident simulations can help staff to react effectively and quickly in the event of a real emergency.

Chapter 13:
INNOVATIONS AND NEW TECHNIQUES

The development of radiopharmaceuticals.

The evolution of radiopharmaceuticals is an exciting tale of innovation and scientific advances that have reshaped the landscape of nuclear medicine over the decades. Radiopharmaceuticals are specific compounds which, when labelled with radionuclides, can be used to obtain diagnostic images or deliver targeted treatment. The history of their development is closely linked to advances in chemistry, physics and biology.

1. The beginnings :
In the 1950s and 1960s, with the discovery of new radioactive isotopes, the first radiopharmaceuticals were introduced. Iodine-131, for example, rapidly became a valuable tool for the diagnosis and treatment of thyroid disease.

2. Development of imaging techniques :
With the advent of scintigraphy in the 1970s, the demand for radiopharmaceuticals suitable for imaging increased. Technetium-99m, because of its ideal half-life and radiological properties, became the most widely used isotope for scintigraphy.

3. Personalised radiopharmaceuticals :
In the 1980s and 1990s, research focused on creating specific molecules that could target particular cells or biological processes, paving the way for more personalised and targeted nuclear medicine.

4. The era of theranostics :
Since the 2000s, the fusion of the words "therapy" and "diagnosis" has given rise to "theranostics". This refers to

the use of radiopharmaceuticals that can both diagnose and treat a disease, often with the same compound. Radiopeptide treatments, such as lutetium-177 DOTATATE for certain neuroendocrine tumours, are examples of this.

5. Radiopharmaceuticals for neurology :

The development of radiopharmaceuticals for brain imaging, particularly for diagnosing diseases such as Alzheimer's, has evolved significantly. Compounds capable of targeting amyloid plaques or the tau protein have revolutionised the way these diseases are diagnosed and studied.

6. Recent innovations and outlook :

With advances in technology and a growing understanding of molecular biology, today's radiopharmaceuticals are more targeted, effective and safe. Current research is focusing on the development of radionuclide therapies for various types of cancer, as well as improving the detection of disease at an early stage.

Radiopharmaceuticals have come a long way from their beginnings as simple diagnostic tools to powerful therapeutic agents. As research advances, we can expect to see revolutionary new radiopharmaceuticals that will offer new treatment and diagnostic opportunities for many diseases.

Technological advances in imaging.

Technological advances in medical imaging have transformed the way doctors diagnose, treat and monitor disease. Nuclear medicine, in particular, has benefited from these innovations, opening up new ways of treating patients. In this tour, we will explore the advances that have been made and the impact they have had on medical practice.

From the outset, the fusion of physics, chemistry and biology laid the foundations for medical imaging. But it was with the rise of computing and digital technology that medical imaging really took off.

1. The digital age :
The transition from analogue to digital imaging marked a revolution. Not only are digital images of superior quality, they can also be easily stored, shared and analysed. The introduction of computed tomography (CT) in the 1970s, which uses X-rays to obtain sliced images of the body, is a perfect example.

2. The advent of MRI :
Magnetic Resonance Imaging (MRI) has changed the game by making it possible to visualise soft tissue as never before. Without using ionising radiation, MRI uses a powerful magnetic field to obtain detailed images, opening up new perspectives for analysing the brain, joints and other organs.

3. PET and PET-CT :
Positron emission tomography (PET) has opened a window onto the molecular biology of the human body. By combining PET with CT, doctors can now obtain both anatomical and functional information, enabling precise localisation and characterisation of lesions.

4. Interventional radiology :
Advances in real-time imaging make it possible to perform minimally invasive surgery under radiological guidance, reducing risks and speeding up recovery.

5. Artificial intelligence and machine learning :
These technologies offer fascinating possibilities for image analysis and interpretation. They can help to identify complex pathologies, precisely quantify certain features and predict clinical outcomes from large image databases.

6. Molecular imaging and multimodality :
The integration of different imaging modalities offers a complete and holistic view of the patient. For example, combining MRI and PET scans provides additional information on anatomy and function.

7. Three-dimensional imaging and augmented reality :
The ability to visualise complex body structures in 3D, and even to superimpose them using augmented reality during operations, represents enormous potential for surgery and other medical procedures.

Technological advances in medical imaging have shaped and continue to reshape the landscape of nuclear medicine. These innovations, coupled with ongoing research and the adaptability of healthcare professionals, ensure that imaging will play a central role in the future of patient care.

Future prospects nuclear medicine.

Nuclear medicine, with its unique diagnostic and therapeutic applications, has established itself as an essential pillar of modern medicine. As we look to the future, it is clear that the combination of research, technological innovation and clinical demand will continue to push the boundaries of this field. Let's take a look at the future prospects for nuclear medicine.

1. Targeted therapies :
The future of nuclear medicine is intrinsically linked to the development of radionuclide therapies. Targeted treatments, using specific isotopes to attack cancer cells while sparing healthy tissue, are enjoying remarkable growth. Research is focusing on the development of more

specific agents, capable of precisely targeting different forms of cancer.

2. Hybrid imaging :
The combination of imaging modalities, such as PET-CT or PET-MRI, will continue to improve, offering greater resolution and specificity. These hybrid systems enable better localisation, characterisation and assessment of diseases.

3. Personalised care :
In the era of personalised medicine, nuclear medicine will play a key role in the development of tailor-made treatments. Patients could benefit from individualised therapeutic approaches based on their genetics, physiology and the biology of their disease.

4. Artificial intelligence (AI) :
AI is set to revolutionise nuclear medicine diagnostics. It can help improve accuracy, reduce errors, and provide more in-depth analyses of images, going beyond what the human eye can perceive.

5. New-generation radiopharmaceuticals :
With advances in medicinal chemistry and molecular biology, new radiopharmaceuticals will emerge, offering greater specificity, reduced radiation dose and improved biodistribution.

6. Training and education :
With the rapid evolution of the field, continuing education will be essential. Educational programmes will need to adapt to new technologies and therapies, ensuring that healthcare professionals remain at the cutting edge of clinical practice.

7. Interdisciplinary collaboration :
Nuclear medicine will strengthen its collaboration with other disciplines, including oncology, cardiology, neurology and surgery, to provide integrated patient care.

8. Ethical and regulatory issues :
With the adoption of new technologies and therapies, new ethical and regulatory issues will emerge, requiring an open and informed dialogue between professionals, regulators and the public.

Nuclear medicine is at the dawn of an exciting era. With a combination of advanced technology, innovative research and growing clinical demand, the field is well placed to continue improving the lives of patients around the world.

Chapter 14:
COMMUNICATION
WITH FAMILIES AND FRIENDS

Inform without alarm:
the delicate equation.

Communicating with the families and loved ones of nuclear medicine patients is a subtle art that oscillates between the need to inform and the need to reassure. In a context where the terms 'radioactivity' or 'radiation' can evoke irrational fears or memories of historic incidents, the challenge for healthcare professionals is to demystify the process while providing clear, factual information.

When a patient has to undergo a nuclear medicine examination or treatment, their family may naturally feel anxious, amplified by a lack of understanding. Technical terms and procedures can seem intimidating to those unfamiliar with the field. This is where the crucial role of healthcare staff comes into play, particularly nurses, who are often on the front line in answering questions and allaying concerns.

The first step in this communication is active listening. It is essential to understand the specific concerns of each family, as this enables communication to be targeted to meet their needs directly. One family may fear potential side effects, while another may worry about the length of time they will be exposed to radiation.

Once these concerns have been identified, it is essential to provide accurate information, but also to present it in a way that is both accessible and reassuring. It's not just about bombarding the family with facts, but contextualising them.

For example, rather than simply saying that a certain dose of radiation is 'safe', it can be useful to compare it with everyday exposures, such as a plane flight or a dental X-ray, to give perspective.

It is also crucial to acknowledge and validate families' feelings. Minimising their concerns or dismissing them out of hand can leave them feeling unvalidated or misunderstood. Instead, it is beneficial to adopt an empathetic approach, acknowledging their concerns while providing clarification.

Finally, patience is essential. Everyone assimilates information at their own pace, and some families may need several explanations or reassurances before they feel comfortable.

Communicating with families and loved ones in nuclear medicine is a delicate dance between information and compassion. By approaching each interaction with empathy, patience and clarity, healthcare professionals can transform concern into understanding and fear into confidence.

The nurse's support role.

The support role of the nurse goes well beyond direct clinical care. In nuclear medicine, as in other medical fields, the nurse is often the first point of contact for patients and their families. They are the human face in the midst of sophisticated machines and potentially intimidating treatments. It's a role that requires a combination of technical expertise, communication skills and deep empathy.

Nurses guide patients through their medical journey
When patients arrive for an examination or treatment, they can be overwhelmed by the unknown. Nurses break down the steps, explain procedures, answer questions and help to dispel any myths or misconceptions the patient may have about radioactivity or the effects of treatment.

The nurse, an emotional pillar
Faced with fear, uncertainty and, in some cases, an alarming diagnosis, patients need emotional support. Nurses offer a listening ear, reassurance, encouragement and, where necessary, referral to specialist professionals such as psychologists or social workers.

Nurses as health educators
An essential part of support is educating the patient about their condition, the potential effects of treatment and how to manage the aftermath. This education is vital not only for the patient's understanding, but also for their adherence to treatment and ability to make informed decisions.

The nurse, intermediary between the patient and the medical team
Nurses often act as intermediaries, relaying the patient's concerns or questions to the medical team, and vice versa. They act as a bridge, ensuring fluid and effective communication for the well-being of the patient.

The nurse, protecting the patient's dignity
At moments of vulnerability, such as when a patient is exposed for a procedure, the nurse ensures that the patient's dignity is preserved, by offering comfort, respecting privacy and responding to individual needs.

The nurse, supporting families
Families may also have questions, fears and needs. Nurses also support relatives, informing and guiding them through the medical process.

The support role of the nuclear medicine nurse is multidimensional. It involves combining technical expertise with empathy, compassion and communication to offer holistic support to both the patient and their loved ones. This role is measured not simply in terms of actions, but in the lasting impact it has on the patient's mental, emotional and physical well-being.

Working with teams psychological support.

In nuclear medicine, collaboration with psychological support teams is of vital importance. Patients are often confronted with complex diagnoses and procedures that can be a source of anxiety. Add to this the weight of common misconceptions about radioactivity, and it's clear that psychological support is essential to ensure patients' well-being.

Assessing the need for psychological support :
From the very first contact, nurses are trained to spot signs of psychological distress. Whether it's anxiety, depression, refusal of treatment or any other emotional reaction, the nurse can recommend a consultation with a mental health professional.

Facilitating communication :
Nurses often act as intermediaries between the patient and the medical team, including psychological support teams. They may help prepare the patient for sessions with a psychologist, clarify the patient's concerns or simply act as a liaison to ensure that the patient receives the necessary support.

Education and awareness :
Nurses work closely with the psychological support teams to educate patients about the benefits of taking charge of

their mental health. They may also co-facilitate workshops or information sessions on topics such as stress management, relaxation or meditation.

Integrative strategies :

The nurse and the psychological support team can work together to integrate stress management strategies into the patient's care plan, such as deep breathing, visualisation or even meditation techniques.

Coordinated responses to crises :

In situations where the patient is in severe distress or crisis, a rapid and coordinated response is crucial. The nurse may work with psychologists, psychiatrists and other mental health professionals to ensure that the patient receives immediate and appropriate care.

Exchanging information and knowledge :

Collaboration between nurses and psychological support teams is not one-way. It is also essential for nurses to inform psychologists about the particularities of nuclear medicine, so that they can adapt their support accordingly.

Follow-up:

After a procedure or treatment, the nurse continues to monitor the patient's psychological well-being, ensuring that they have access to the necessary resources and adjusting the care plan as required.

The collaboration between nuclear medicine nurses and psychological support teams is a synergy that aims to envelop the patient in holistic care, taking into account not only their physical needs, but also their emotional and mental well-being. In a field as specialised and often misunderstood as nuclear medicine, this collaboration is essential to ensure an optimal patient experience.

Chapter 15:
THE CHALLENGES OF IT
AND TELEMEDICINE

Electronic file management
and data integrity.

In the modern healthcare landscape, electronic records management and data integrity have become major concerns. For the nuclear medicine nurse, this is no exception. Electronic records offer a host of advantages over traditional paper records, particularly in terms of accessibility, efficiency and communication between healthcare professionals. However, they also bring new challenges in terms of confidentiality, security and data integrity.
Transition from paper to electronic :

With the advent of hospital information systems and electronic health records (EHRs), many institutions have begun the transition from paper records to digitised versions. This step has required extensive training for nurses in order to master the use of these new systems while guaranteeing the accuracy and confidentiality of patient information.

Accessibility and efficiency :
EHRs have made access to patient information faster and more efficient. A nurse can now consult a patient's medical history, prescribed medicines, allergies, diagnostic images and other relevant data with just a few clicks. This centralisation also facilitates communication between different departments or medical specialities.

Security and confidentiality :
While the benefits of EHRs are undeniable, they also raise security issues. Patient data is sensitive and must be protected from unauthorised access. Nurses need to be trained in security best practice, such as never leaving a computer open and unattended, and using strong, regularly updated passwords.

Data integrity :
Data integrity is paramount. Nurses, who are on the front line of data entry, must ensure that the information recorded is accurate and true. Even a minor error can have a major impact on a patient's diagnosis or treatment.

Updates and maintenance :
EHR systems are regularly updated to incorporate new features, correct any security flaws or improve the user interface. Nurses therefore need to be aware of these updates and, in some cases, receive additional training to adapt to them.

Communication with patients :
With the development of patient portals, individuals can now access their own medical records, ask questions and book appointments online. Nurses may need to guide patients through the use of these portals, or respond to their concerns about the security of their data.

In today's digital world, electronic record management and data integrity are essential skills for any healthcare professional, including nuclear medicine nurses. By ensuring that these systems are used efficiently, securely and ethically, nurses play a key role in guaranteeing optimal patient care.

Telemedicine : opportunities and challenges.

Telemedicine, the remote medical practice that uses information and communication technologies, has expanded rapidly in recent years. While it offers many opportunities, particularly in terms of accessibility and cost, it also presents challenges. For nuclear medicine nurses, as for all healthcare professionals, it is essential to understand these two facets in order to best integrate telemedicine into their daily practice.

Telemedicine opportunities :
1. Accessibility :
Telemedicine makes it possible to provide medical care to people who would not otherwise have access to it, particularly those living in rural or remote areas. For nuclear medicine, this can mean providing preliminary consultations or follow-up after an examination or treatment.

2. Continuity of care :
The ability to consult remotely ensures continuity of care, even when the patient or professional is unable to travel. This is particularly relevant in emergency situations or during health crises.

3. Time and cost savings :
Reducing the need for physical travel can generate substantial savings for patients and the healthcare system. It can also increase the number of patients a nurse or doctor can see in a day.

4. Education and training :
Telemedicine can also serve as an educational platform for healthcare professionals, with webinars, online training and exchanges with specialists in various fields.

The challenges of telemedicine :
1. Technological barriers :
Not all patients have access to reliable technology or a stable Internet connection. It is therefore crucial to ensure that these services are accessible to all.

2. Confidentiality and data security :
Online consultations must be secure to protect the confidentiality of medical information. Training nurses and other professionals in best security practices is therefore essential.

3. Regulatory and legal aspects :
Telemedicine raises a number of legal issues, including liability in the event of errors, inter-state or international professional licences, and insurance reimbursement.

4. Clinical limitations :
Some aspects of the physical examination cannot be carried out remotely. Furthermore, in nuclear medicine, while consultations can be carried out remotely, examinations require a physical presence.

5. Human relations :
Telemedicine can potentially diminish the human aspect of the care-giver-patient relationship. It is therefore crucial to find ways of maintaining warm, empathetic communication, even through a screen.

While telemedicine offers incredible opportunities to improve the accessibility and efficiency of care, it also presents challenges that require constant reflection and adaptation. For nuclear medicine nurses, the important thing is to embrace these new technologies while ensuring that the quality and safety of care is maintained.

Ensuring the confidentiality and security of patient information.

Ensuring the confidentiality and security of patient information is a cornerstone of medical practice and fundamental to building a relationship of trust between patient and healthcare professional. For the nuclear medicine nurse, as for any other healthcare professional, this responsibility is essential. With the emergence of information technologies in medicine, this mission is taking on an even more critical dimension.

Protecting sensitive information :
Every consultation, examination and interaction in nuclear medicine generates a wealth of information about the patient. This information may include personal data, medical images, medical histories and other sensitive details. Disclosure of this information could not only violate the patient's right to privacy, but also leave him or her vulnerable to malicious acts.

Measures to guarantee confidentiality and security :
1. Secure electronic systems :
The use of encrypted medical information systems protected by complex passwords is essential. Regular updates and the use of firewalls can also help protect against cyber attacks.

2. Access protocols :
Only healthcare professionals involved in the patient's care should have access to his or her information. The use of badges or access cards, as well as two-factor identification protocols, can limit unauthorised access.

3. Continuing education :
Healthcare professionals, including nuclear medicine nurses, must receive regular training on confidentiality and

information security. This includes information on the latest threats, as well as best practice for protecting patient data.

4. Secure destruction :
When patient information is no longer required, it must be securely destroyed. For paper documents, this means appropriate shredding. For electronic data, this requires deletion methods that render the data irretrievable.

5. Informed consent :
Patients must be informed of how their information is used and stored. They must also give their consent for any sharing of information with third parties.

6. Secure communication :
When patient information is shared between healthcare professionals, secure communication channels, such as encrypted emails or VPN connections, must be used.

Trust is an essential element of the patient-healthcare provider relationship, and the protection of patient information is at the heart of this trust. Nuclear medicine nurses, working in a field where technology plays such a central role, have a particular responsibility to ensure that every stage, from booking the appointment to carrying out the examination and follow-up, scrupulously respects the confidentiality and security of patient information.

Chapter 16:
THE ROLE OF THE NURSE
IN EDUCATION AND TRAINING

Educating patients :
understanding for better acceptance.

In the complex world of nuclear medicine, nurses often find themselves at the intersection between advanced technology and anxious patients. Faced with technical terms such as "scintigraphy" or "radiopharmaceutical", the latter may feel lost or even frightened. This is where patient education comes in, an essential process for enlightening, reassuring and involving patients in their care.

Despite its prodigious advances, nuclear medicine remains shrouded in an aura of mystery for the general public. Images of atoms and radiation, often associated with danger in the collective imagination, can be a source of concern. However, when patients understand how the procedure works, its benefits and the relative risks involved, they are able to see beyond their initial apprehensions.

Education starts with simplification. Nurses, with their empathetic approach, are perfectly placed to translate medical jargon into understandable terms. Explaining that a radiopharmaceutical is simply a substance that enables certain parts of the body to be visualised, or that a scintigraphy is nothing more than a special camera that detects these substances, can make a huge difference.
But beyond simplification, it is crucial to establish a dialogue. Encouraging patients to ask questions, express their fears and share their concerns helps to build a relationship of trust. Only by truly understanding the

patient's concerns can the nurse provide relevant and reassuring information.

Education also plays a crucial role in the preparation and follow-up of procedures. A patient who is well informed about what to expect before, during and after a procedure will be better able to follow instructions, which can greatly improve results and minimise the risk of side effects or complications.

Educating patients in nuclear medicine is not just a matter of passing on information. It's a process that aims to empower patients, transforming them from passive recipients of care into active players in their own health. And when a patient understands and accepts a procedure, they not only have a more positive experience, they are also more likely to adhere to medical recommendations, which increases the chances of a successful outcome.

Training new members of the team.

Welcoming new members to a nuclear medicine team is not just a matter of passing on technical knowledge. It's also about sharing the department's culture, values and mission, and ensuring that each new recruit is both competent and in tune with the expectations of the job.

Integration and induction: A new member's first few days in the team are crucial. It's vital to ensure a smooth integration, which involves an introduction to the team, the premises, the equipment and the protocols in place. This introductory phase lays the foundations for a healthy and productive working relationship.

Passing on knowledge: Nuclear medicine is a complex and constantly evolving field. Providing technical training for newcomers is fundamental. This involves both theoretical and practical sessions, where the newcomer can observe, ask questions and finally, under supervision, carry out the tasks assigned to him or her.

Mentoring : Coaching by a mentor, an experienced member of the team, can greatly facilitate integration. The mentor will be the newcomer's point of contact, able to answer their questions, guide them and provide constructive feedback on their performance.

Safety awareness: Handling radioactive isotopes and sophisticated equipment requires a thorough knowledge of safety measures. New members must be rigorously trained in these protocols, not only for their own safety but also for that of patients and the team as a whole.

Continuing education: As nuclear medicine is a rapidly evolving field, training never really stops. It is essential to ensure that new members are aware of this need for continuing education, and that they are encouraged to attend seminars, conferences and other training courses throughout their careers.

Valuing everyone's contribution: A new employee, even if just starting out, brings a fresh perspective and may have innovative ideas. It's essential to value these contributions, and to encourage the exchange of ideas and collaboration between old and new members.

Feedback and evaluation: Finally, to ensure that the training is effective, it is essential to set up regular evaluations to identify strengths and areas for improvement, and to adjust the training accordingly.

Ultimately, training new team members is an ongoing process that aims not only to ensure operational excellence, but also to reinforce team spirit and ensure that each member feels valued, competent and fulfilled in their role.

Take part in conferences and workshops.

At the heart of nuclear medicine lies a dynamic of continuous innovation. Technological advances, scientific discoveries and new therapeutic protocols are constantly emerging. In this ever-changing environment, attending conferences and workshops is not only a learning opportunity, but also a necessity for any professional wishing to remain at the cutting edge of their field.

1. Broaden your horizons: Conferences, whether national or international, offer a panoramic view of recent advances in the field. Exchanges with peers from different backgrounds allow you to compare your practices, adopt new methods and open up to sometimes radically different approaches.

2. Technical training: The practical workshops, often organised alongside the conferences, are ideal opportunities to familiarise yourself with the latest technologies, learn new techniques or hone your skills under the guidance of recognised experts.

3. Strengthen your professional network: These events are also unique networking opportunities. Forging links with colleagues, researchers, industrialists or other professionals can open the door to fruitful collaborations, career opportunities or even lasting friendships.

4. Contribute to the community: Conferences and workshops are not just places to passively receive information. They are also a platform for sharing your own discoveries, feedback and innovations. Presenting a study, leading a workshop or simply taking an active part in the discussions reinforces the sense of belonging to a professional community.

5. Re-energise and motivate: Beyond the purely professional aspect, these events are often moments of rejuvenation. They offer a break from the daily grind, stimulate motivation and rekindle passion for the job.

6. Ethics and responsibility: Many conferences also address the ethical issues associated with nuclear medicine. In a world where technology sometimes evolves faster than ethical thinking, it is crucial for professionals to consider the implications of their actions.

7. Preparing for the future: Finally, keeping up to date through conferences and workshops helps you to anticipate future trends, prepare for the challenges ahead and make informed career choices.

Taking an active part in conferences and workshops is a multi-faceted investment. It is a process that enriches the professional from a technical, ethical, human and strategic point of view, while contributing to the influence of nuclear medicine throughout the world.

Chapter 17:
QUALITY ISSUES AND ACCREDITATION

Norms and standards
in nuclear medicine.

Nuclear medicine, at the crossroads of biology, physics and medical technology, is a particularly complex and sensitive field. The slightest deviation or inaccuracy can have serious consequences for both patients and healthcare professionals. That's why norms and standards are so important: they are the foundation on which the entire discipline rests, guaranteeing optimum levels of care and safety.

1. The foundations of the standards: These standards were not created ex nihilo. They are the result of intense collaboration between experts in the field, scientists, doctors, technicians and professional associations. They are based on rigorous scientific data, feedback from experience and constant technological monitoring.

2. Safety first and foremost: Nuclear medicine uses radioactive substances and sophisticated equipment. Standards strictly govern their use, minimising the risks of exposure for patients and the medical team. This covers both the preparation and administration of radiopharmaceuticals and the operation and maintenance of the equipment.

3. Harmonised protocols : Established standards enable practices to be harmonised across different institutions and countries. This means that patients receive the same quality of care whether they are in Paris, Tokyo or New York. This uniformity is essential for the comparability of results, the training of professionals and clinical research.

4. Quality assurance: The standards also include quality assurance procedures. This involves regular checks, audits and validations to ensure that current practices comply with established standards. This is a guarantee of confidence for patients and a continuous improvement process for professionals.

5. Adaptability and evolution: The world of nuclear medicine is changing rapidly. New discoveries, technological advances, feedback... all this requires that norms and standards be regularly revised and updated. This adaptability ensures that the discipline remains at the cutting edge of excellence.

6. Shared responsibility: Compliance with standards is everyone's business. Every professional, whether doctor, nurse, technician or administrator, has a role to play in ensuring that standards are met. It's a collective responsibility, a sign of seriousness and commitment to patients.

7. Awareness-raising and training: Adopting the standards requires constant awareness-raising and training of teams. Ongoing training sessions, practical workshops and simulations are essential to ensure that everyone masters the protocols in force.

Norms and standards in nuclear medicine are not simply bureaucratic guidelines. They reflect the deep commitment of an entire community to excellence, safety and the well-being of patients.

Preparing for audits and assessments.

The world of nuclear medicine, with its complex mix of advanced technology, radioactive substances and human interaction, requires constant monitoring to ensure the safety and quality of care. Audits and assessments are essential tools for achieving this objective. Careful preparation is therefore crucial to passing these exams and ensuring a working environment that meets established standards.

1. Understanding the objectives of the audit: First and foremost, it is essential to understand the purpose of the audit. Is it an internal audit or is it mandated by an external entity? Is it focused on safety, quality of care, regulatory compliance or a combination of these? Knowing the objectives will enable you to target your preparations effectively.

2. Putting together a dedicated team: Bringing together an interdisciplinary team, including representatives from all the sectors concerned (doctors, nurses, technicians, administrators), will make it easier to coordinate efforts and ensure that all aspects of practice are examined.

3. Document review: Ensure that all protocols, manuals, registers and patient records are up to date and easily accessible. Documents must reflect the day-to-day reality of operations and comply with current standards.

4. Simulations and practical exercises: Organising mock audits can help the team to identify areas of risk and get used to the assessment process. It also builds confidence and reduces the anxiety associated with the actual audit.

5. Staff training and awareness: Each member of the team must be aware of their responsibilities and the procedures to be followed. Regular training sessions and reminders will ensure that everyone is compliant and prepared.

6. Analysis of previous incidents: Previous incidents, whether minor or major, can offer valuable lessons. They should be analysed in detail to avoid their recurrence and to demonstrate the capacity for continuous improvement.

7. Prepare the equipment : All equipment, whether gamma cameras, PET scanners or other machines, must be in perfect working order, correctly calibrated and maintained.

8. Open communication: Encouraging a culture of open communication within the team is essential. Everyone should feel free to express their concerns, suggestions or questions.

9. Post-audit feedback: Once the audit has been completed, it is essential to bring the team together to discuss the results, strengths and areas for improvement. This stage is crucial to the positive development of the service.

10. Action plan: On the basis of the audit observations and recommendations, draw up a clear action plan, with precise deadlines, to rectify the shortcomings identified.

Preparing for audits and assessments in nuclear medicine is an ongoing process, requiring constant involvement and vigilance. This is the price we have to pay to ensure that our practice is optimised, safe and compliant with the most demanding standards.

Continuous improvement initiatives.

In the world of healthcare, the adage "The only constant is change" has never been truer. In nuclear medicine, where technology, regulations and patient needs are constantly evolving, the quest for excellence is a never-ending journey. Adopting a continuous improvement approach is not only desirable, it's essential. It means always questioning, evaluating and optimising current practices to offer the best possible quality of care.

1. Cultivate a culture of improvement: The first step to success is to instil a mindset where continuous improvement is valued and encouraged. This means promoting a culture where questioning is seen not as criticism, but as an opportunity for growth.

2. Feedback: The implementation of feedback systems, where incidents, whether minor or major, are analysed to learn lessons from them, is fundamental. These lessons can be used to adapt protocols and avoid repeating the same mistakes.

3. Regular training: Nuclear medicine is a field in which innovations are frequent. Regular staff training is essential if we are to keep abreast of the latest advances and guarantee optimum patient care.

4. Process evaluation: A regular review of the processes in place, from examination protocols to communication methods, enables areas for optimisation to be identified. Methods such as Lean Healthcare can be adopted to streamline operations and improve efficiency.

5. Interdisciplinary collaboration: Improvement does not happen in silos. Collaborating with other disciplines, whether radiology, oncology or surgery, offers a broader perspective and enables us to benefit from collective expertise.

6. Patient feedback: Who better than patients to provide valuable information on the quality of care? Their feedback, whether positive or negative, is an invaluable source of information for improving the patient experience.

7. Use of technology: The adoption of new technological tools, whether advanced imaging equipment or information systems, can greatly improve the accuracy of diagnosis and the effectiveness of treatment.

8. Audit and certification: Subjecting the service to regular external audits or certification can provide an objective assessment of current practices and suggest areas for improvement.

9. Scientific watch: Keeping abreast of the latest research, studies and publications in the field ensures that practice is based on the most up-to-date evidence.

10. Pilot projects: Testing new methods or approaches on a small scale enables us to assess their effectiveness before rolling them out more widely.

Continuous improvement in nuclear medicine is a proactive, dynamic and collaborative approach. It aims to constantly push back the boundaries of excellence to guarantee the highest possible quality of care, with respect for patients and professionals alike.

Chapter 18:
NURSES AND INTERNATIONAL COLLABORATION

Exchanges and collaboration with foreign centres.

In this age of globalisation, collaboration and exchanges with centres abroad play a crucial role in the development and evolution of nuclear medicine. More than ever, knowledge and skills are crossing borders, enriching medical practices around the world. International collaborations open up new perspectives, pave the way for innovation and enhance the quality of patient care.

1. The benefits of diversity: Working with foreign centres offers a unique opportunity to discover different working methods, varied clinical approaches and innovative technologies. Each country and culture has its own specific characteristics which can enrich the overall understanding of the discipline.

2. Sharing knowledge: International conferences, workshops and seminars are valuable platforms for exchanging expertise, discussing complex cases and disseminating new techniques or discoveries.

3. Exchange programmes: These initiatives enable professionals, whether doctors, technicians or nurses, to spend a period of time in a foreign centre to develop their skills, share their knowledge and adopt new methodologies.

4. Joint research : International collaboration makes it easier to set up joint research projects, drawing on the resources and expertise of several institutions to tackle complex issues.

5. Standardisation and harmonisation: Working closely with international centres allows us to harmonise practices and move towards standardisation of protocols, guaranteeing optimum quality and safety for patients, wherever in the world they may be.

6. Technological development: Innovation in nuclear medicine is constantly evolving. Collaboration with leading centres abroad can accelerate the adoption of new technologies, offering cutting-edge care to patients.

7. Training and education: International collaborations encourage the setting up of joint training programmes, internships and residencies abroad, providing valuable experience for future professionals in the field.

8. Crisis management: In exceptional situations, such as isotope shortages or global events affecting nuclear medicine, strong cooperation between foreign centres can make it easier to find solutions and pool resources.

9. Ethics and regulation: Exchanges with international centres help to compare and harmonise ethical and regulatory approaches, ensuring better protection for patients and a practice that complies with global standards.

10. Strengthening diplomatic ties: In addition to the medical and scientific benefits, collaboration in nuclear medicine can strengthen diplomatic ties between countries, fostering a climate of trust and cooperation.

Exchanges and collaborations with foreign nuclear medicine centres are a valuable opportunity. They help to enrich knowledge, improve practices and provide the best possible quality of care to patients around the world. In an interconnected world, collaboration is the key to progress.

Understanding the different approaches to nuclear medicine around the world.

Nuclear medicine, although based on universal scientific principles, has adapted and evolved differently in different parts of the world. Influenced by factors such as access to technology, specific health needs, medical traditions, economics and regulation, each region offers a unique perspective on the application and development of this medical speciality.

1. The West : Pioneers and innovators
   - North America and Europe were pioneers in the development and application of nuclear medicine. With significant investment in research and development, these regions introduced many of the standardised technologies and protocols used today.
   - Challenges such as an ageing population have led to an increase in heart and neurological diseases, making nuclear medicine a crucial tool for diagnosis and monitoring.
2. Asia: Rapid growth and innovative approaches
   - Countries such as Japan, South Korea and China quickly adopted and adapted nuclear medicine, sometimes developing their own technologies and methods.
   - Medical traditions such as traditional Chinese medicine can influence the diagnostic and therapeutic approach.
3. Africa: Potential and challenges
   - While access to nuclear medicine remains limited in many parts of Africa, initiatives to extend this speciality are underway.
   - Endemic diseases such as malaria could benefit from new diagnostic approaches thanks to nuclear medicine.

4. Latin America: Balancing tradition and technology
   - With increasing adoption of nuclear medicine, countries such as Brazil and Argentina are playing a leading role in the region.
   - Specific health needs, such as tropical diseases, influence the applications of nuclear medicine.
5. Middle East: an intersection of tradition and modernity
   - The Middle East, rich in oil resources, is investing more and more in cutting-edge medical care, including nuclear medicine.
   - Combining traditional medical practices with modern technologies offers a unique perspective.
6. Oceania: Access and specific geographical features
   - The vast distances in Australia and New Zealand present challenges in terms of access to healthcare.
   - Nuclear medicine plays a key role in remote diagnosis and telemedicine.

Nuclear medicine has evolved in many different ways around the world, anchored in a variety of cultural, economic and health contexts. Understanding these diverse approaches not only enriches the global perspective of the specialty, but also paves the way for innovations and international collaborations that benefit us all.

Exchange programmes and training abroad.

In the constantly evolving field of nuclear medicine, globalisation offers invaluable opportunities for healthcare professionals to train, share knowledge and collaborate across borders. Exchange and training programmes abroad play an essential role in this dynamic exchange, contributing to the advancement of the discipline worldwide.

1. The importance of international trade
    They offer exposure to new methods, technologies and approaches in nuclear medicine.
    They provide a better understanding of the challenges and solutions adopted by other cultures and healthcare systems.
2. Types of programmes available
    Clinical placements: Nurses and doctors can spend time in foreign hospitals, learning directly from their international counterparts.
    Academic training: These programmes are often linked to academic institutions and lead to diplomas or certifications.
    Workshops and seminars: Organised around specific subjects, these provide intensive training in a short space of time.
3. Benefits for professionals
    Expanding skills: Learning techniques and protocols that may be different from those practised in the home country.
    Networking: Create lasting links with professionals from all over the world.
    Cultural perspective: Understanding how cultural differences can influence the approach to care.
4. Challenges and how to overcome them
    Language barriers: It is essential to be proficient in the language of the host country or to be trained in a common language.
    Regulatory differences: Standards and regulations may vary from one country to another. It is crucial to find out before starting a programme.
5. The role of international organisations
    Bodies such as the International Atomic Energy Agency (IAEA) and the European Society of Nuclear Medicine (EANM) offer programmes, resources and grants to encourage international exchanges.

6. How to maximise the experience

Preparation: Find out all you can about the country, the culture and the specific medical requirements of the region.

Active engagement: Actively participate in training, ask questions and interact with local colleagues.

Sharing after return: Pass on the knowledge you have acquired to colleagues in your home country.

Exchange and training programmes abroad represent a unique opportunity for nuclear medicine professionals to enrich themselves both professionally and personally. In an increasingly connected world, these exchanges encourage innovation, collaboration and the advancement of nuclear medicine for the benefit of all.

Chapter 19:
LEGAL ASPECTS AND ETHICS IN NUCLEAR MEDICINE

Nurses' legal responsibilities.

Nuclear medicine, as a medical discipline that uses radioactive substances to diagnose, treat and research disease, presents unique ethical and legal challenges. For nurses working in this field, understanding the legal and ethical implications is essential.

1. Administration of radiopharmaceuticals
The administration of radioactive substances requires not only specialist training, but also a thorough understanding of the associated risks. Nurses are legally obliged to administer the correct dose, monitor side effects and document any incidents.

2. Radiological protection
Safety is paramount. Nurses have a legal responsibility to protect the patient, themselves and the medical team from excessive radiation. This involves knowledge of shielding techniques, the safe storage of radioactive substances and the monitoring of radiation exposure.

3. Informed consent
Before any nuclear medicine procedure, the patient must be fully informed of the risks and benefits. The nurse plays a key role in this process, ensuring that the patient understands and gives informed consent.

4. Confidentiality
As in all medical fields, nuclear medicine nurses are bound by professional secrecy. However, given the sensitive nature of the examinations and treatments, particular attention must be paid to protecting patient information.

5. Ethical research

Nuclear medicine is also a rapidly evolving area of research. When nurses take part in clinical studies, they must be aware of ethical standards, particularly with regard to participant consent and full disclosure of risks.

6. Ongoing training

Nuclear medicine technology and techniques evolve rapidly. Nurses are legally obliged to keep their skills up to date in order to guarantee safe and effective care.

7. Managing radioactive waste

The nurse's legal responsibility does not end with the administration of treatment. They must also be aware of the procedures for managing radioactive waste and materials to ensure everyone's safety.

8. Interdisciplinary collaboration

Working closely with nuclear medicine physicians, technologists and other health professionals, nurses must know the limits of their skills and when to consult or refer a patient to a specialist.

Nuclear medicine, while offering exciting opportunities for care and research, also presents unique legal and ethical challenges. The nurse, as an essential member of the healthcare team, must carefully and competently navigate this complex landscape to ensure the safety and well-being of patients.

Common ethical dilemmas.

Nuclear medicine, like all medical disciplines, is faced with ethical dilemmas. Although this speciality offers undeniable advantages in terms of diagnosis and treatment, it also raises specific concerns due to the use of radiation and radioactive substances. Here are some of the ethical dilemmas commonly encountered:

1. Risk versus benefit

At the heart of medicine lies the principle of "do no harm". But when it comes to using radiation, how do you balance the potential benefit of an accurate diagnosis or effective treatment with the potential risk associated with radiation exposure?

2. Informed consent

Even if patients are informed of the risks and benefits, do they really understand the nature and scope of the procedures? Ensuring that patients not only consent, but fully understand, is a constant challenge.

3. Use of research

Nuclear medicine is a rapidly evolving discipline with new discoveries. However, using a new and unproven technology or technique raises ethical issues, particularly when considering the implications for the patient.

4. Equitable access to care

With limited resources, including rare isotopes, how can we ensure equitable access to treatment and diagnosis? Who should have priority and on what basis?

5. Protection of privacy

The images produced by nuclear medicine may reveal information about other aspects of the patient's health. To what extent should these incidental findings be shared with the patient or other healthcare professionals?

6. Managing radioactive waste

Ethical responsibility does not end with the administration of treatment. How can the waste produced be managed ethically and safely, with due regard for the environment and future generations?

7. Training and competence

Professionals must be properly trained to use nuclear medicine technologies. However, with the rapid evolution of technology, how can we ensure that professionals remain competent and up to date?

8. Transparency in the event of an error

If an error occurs, such as an incorrect dose being

administered, how should this be communicated to the patient? What is the ethical responsibility to the patient in such cases?

9. Interprofessional collaboration
Collaboration between different medical specialties is essential to ensure the best patient care. However, it can also lead to tensions or conflicts of interest. How are these situations handled ethically?

Every ethical dilemma in nuclear medicine requires careful thought, putting the interests of the patient first, while balancing the longer-term implications for society and the environment. The key lies in solid ethical training, transparent communication and constant updating of knowledge and skills.

Major legal cases
that have influenced practice.

Nuclear medicine, being a speciality at the cutting edge of medical technology, is not free from controversy and litigation. While some countries may have specific cases that have influenced their legislation or guidelines, here are some general themes of court cases that could have an impact on practice:

Accidental radiation exposure: These cases involve patients who have accidentally received excessive doses of radiation during diagnosis or treatment. The health implications of such errors can be serious, and these cases have led to large claims for compensation, forcing medical facilities to strengthen their safety protocols.

Non-disclosure of risks: This may involve situations where the patient has not been sufficiently informed of the potential risks associated with a nuclear medicine treatment or diagnosis, leading to allegations of failure to obtain informed consent.

Diagnostic errors: As in other medical specialities, diagnostic errors in nuclear medicine can have serious repercussions on a patient's health. These cases can lead to allegations of medical negligence.

Radioactive waste management: Medical facilities can be sued for poor management of radioactive waste, particularly if this leads to environmental contamination or employee exposure.

Worker exposure: Healthcare professionals working in the field of nuclear medicine are exposed to a radiation risk. If safety protocols are not properly followed, this can lead to unnecessary exposure, resulting in legal action.

Equipment safety incidents: Machine failures or calibration errors can result in inappropriate radiation exposures for patients or workers, which can lead to litigation.

Confidentiality issues: As with all medical specialities, unauthorised disclosure of patient information is a major source of litigation.

Unproven technological innovations: Introducing new technologies or treatments into nuclear medicine without appropriate testing can lead to complications for patients, with legal implications for practitioners and hospitals.

These cases have helped to shape legislation, guidelines and best practice in nuclear medicine, focusing on patient safety, proper training of professionals and the implementation of strict protocols to minimise risks.

Chapter 20:
ECOLOGICAL PERSPECTIVES
AND SUSTAINABILITY

Responsible management radiological waste.

Managing radiological waste is an essential part of nuclear medicine. It ensures the safety of patients, healthcare professionals and the environment. Here is a detailed overview of this crucial issue.

Nuclear medicine, with its use of radiopharmaceuticals, generates radioactive waste. This waste may come from the products injected into patients, but also from the materials used to prepare and administer these products, such as syringes, gloves and protective clothing. Responsible management is essential to ensure optimum safety.

Waste classification
Radiological waste is classified according to its nature and radioactive lifetime. These include :
    Short-lived waste, which rapidly loses its radioactivity.
    Long-lived waste, which remains radioactive for long periods.

Storage and disposal
    On-site storage: Short-lived waste can often be stored on the hospital or clinic site until it has lost its radioactivity. This requires special facilities with thick walls to prevent any radiation escaping.
    External disposal: Long-lived waste, on the other hand, must be processed by specialised facilities,

which can store it safely for the time needed for it to decay radioactively.

Reducing waste

Optimising procedures: By using the minimum necessary quantities of radioactive materials and optimising protocols, it is possible to reduce the amount of waste produced.

Recycling: Some elements, such as the lead used for protection, can be recycled after a period of storage.

Training and awareness-raising

All staff working in nuclear medicine must be trained in good practice in the management of radiological waste. This not only ensures their own safety, but also that of their colleagues, patients and the environment.

Safety measures

Strict safety measures must be in place to avoid any accidents. These include the use of suitable containers, the wearing of personal protective equipment, regular monitoring of radiation levels and the establishment of clear protocols in the event of an incident.

Environmental responsibility

Beyond simply complying with regulations, responsible management of radiological waste reflects a medical institution's commitment to environmental protection and public safety.

Managing radiological waste in nuclear medicine is a complex task that requires careful planning, rigorous training and constant monitoring. It is a fundamental part of the professional ethos in nuclear medicine and demonstrates the ongoing commitment of healthcare professionals to ensuring the well-being of all.

Reducing the service's carbon footprint.

Nuclear medicine, although focused on medical diagnosis and treatment, is not exempt from contemporary environmental responsibilities. In the current context of heightened awareness of climate issues, it is crucial for every medical department to adopt an eco-responsible approach. Here are a few ways of reducing the carbon footprint of a nuclear medicine department.

Reducing the carbon footprint starts with an understanding of the entire life cycle of medical procedures, from the equipment used to the waste produced.

Equipment and consumables

Energy-efficient equipment: Modern manufacturers of medical equipment, such as gamma cameras and PET scanners, are developing more energy-efficient machines. Opting for such equipment can significantly reduce energy consumption.

Recycling and reuse: Instead of systematically disposing of consumables after use, consider recycling or sterilisation options for reuse where possible and safe.

Waste management

Minimising waste: Thorough staff training can help to reduce unnecessary waste by avoiding wastage of materials.

Recycling non-radioactive waste: Ensure that waste that is not contaminated by radiopharmaceuticals is correctly sorted and recycled.

Building and infrastructure

Energy-efficient design: Buildings can be designed or renovated to maximise energy efficiency, such as the use of LED lighting, better insulation and efficient heating/cooling systems.

Renewable energy: Consider installing solar panels or other renewable energy sources to power the service.

Mobility and logistics

Transport of radiopharmaceuticals: Optimise logistics to reduce unnecessary journeys, and consider grouping deliveries.

Staff mobility: Encourage environmentally-friendly modes of transport among staff, such as car-sharing, cycling or public transport.

Awareness-raising and training

Environmental education: Provide regular training for staff on the importance of reducing carbon footprints and the best practices to adopt.

Sharing initiatives: Encourage the sharing of eco-responsible ideas and initiatives within the department to continually innovate in energy-efficient practices.

By integrating these methods and adopting a proactive mindset, nuclear medicine departments can play a significant role in the fight against climate change, while offering quality care to their patients.

Promoting an approach eco-responsible within the team.

In a world increasingly aware of environmental issues, promoting an eco-responsible approach in a medical environment such as nuclear medicine is not only a necessity but also a responsibility. Here's how to instil an eco-responsible culture within the nuclear medicine team.

Every member of the team, whether a doctor, nurse, technician or administrator, has a role to play in implementing an eco-responsible approach.

1. Awareness-raising and training

Eco-responsible workshops: Organise in-house seminars or training courses on eco-responsible best practice specific to nuclear medicine.

Regular updates: Provide regular information on the environmental impact of certain common practices and the alternatives available.

2. Establishing clear guidelines

Internal policies: Develop internal policies that encourage eco-responsible practices, such as reducing energy consumption or minimising waste.

Ecological checklists: Create checklists for common procedures, highlighting the steps that can be carried out in a more environmentally-friendly way.

3. Encouraging innovation

Employee suggestions: Encourage staff to suggest ideas to make the service greener and recognise significant contributions.

Managing green projects: Implement pilot projects to test new, more environmentally-friendly methods or technologies.

4. Promoting green mobility

Car-sharing schemes: Encourage staff to share journeys to reduce their carbon footprint.

Incentives for eco-responsible transport: Offer benefits or rewards to employees who opt for environmentally-friendly means of transport, such as cycling or public transport.

5. Accountability

Green managers: Appoint ambassadors or eco-responsible managers within the team to guide and supervise green initiatives.

Audit and feedback: Regularly assess the impact of green initiatives and provide feedback on progress.

6. External collaboration

Green partnerships: Collaborate with other departments or institutions to share best practice and take part in joint green initiatives.

Community involvement: Get involved in local environmental activities to reinforce the team's commitment to sustainability.

Instilling an eco-responsible culture doesn't happen overnight, but with determination, open communication and collective commitment, significant progress can be made. By adopting these measures, the nuclear medicine team is not only protecting the environment, but also reinforcing its mission to treat patients in a way that respects our planet.

Chapter 21:
TRAINING
AND CAREER PROSPECTS

Specialising in nuclear medicine: career paths and training.

Nuclear medicine, at the crossroads of biology, physics and medicine, is a fascinating speciality that has a major impact on the diagnosis and treatment of many diseases. If you're fascinated by the idea of working with radioactive isotopes and using cutting-edge technology to help patients, here's how you can specialise in this field.

1. Basic medical studies

   Initial training: First of all, general medical training is necessary. Most nuclear medicine specialists begin by studying medicine, obtaining the title of Doctor of Medicine.

2. Specialisation in nuclear medicine

   Residency: After medical studies, a residency in nuclear medicine is essential. This post-doctoral training generally lasts between 4 and 5 years, depending on the country, and focuses on clinical practice and the technical aspects of the specialty.

   Certification and accreditation: At the end of residency, it is often necessary to pass an examination or obtain certification to be recognised as a specialist in nuclear medicine.

3. Continuing and further training

   Seminars and workshops: Technology and techniques in nuclear medicine are evolving rapidly. Regular attendance at seminars, workshops and conferences is therefore essential to keep up to date.

Research and development: Many specialists choose to get involved in research to develop new techniques or improve existing methods.

4. Sub-specialities

Nuclear oncology: Focus on the use of nuclear medicine to diagnose and treat cancer.

Nuclear cardiology: Use of nuclear medicine to assess and treat heart disease.

Nuclear endocrinology: Specialising in disorders of the endocrine glands, in particular the thyroid.

5. Complementary skills

Radiation protection training: Essential for working safely with radioactive materials.

Knowledge of medical imaging: For those wishing to focus on scintigraphy or positron emission tomography (PET).

6. Networking and professional affiliations

Membership of professional associations: Membership of nuclear medicine associations or societies can provide opportunities for training, research and networking.

Nuclear medicine is a rich and dynamic speciality. By pursuing a specialist career and engaging in continuing education, you can not only contribute to the advancement of medicine, but also have a profound impact on the lives of many patients.

Career development : management, teaching and research.

Nuclear medicine, like any other medical field, offers a variety of routes for those wishing to progress or diversify their career. Beyond the traditional clinical role, there are opportunities in management, teaching and research to broaden skills, influence clinical practice and contribute to the advancement of science.

1. Management and Leadership

Head of department: Managing a nuclear medicine department involves not only supervising medical staff, but also managing resources, developing policies and taking strategic decisions for the department.

Medical Director: Some professionals gravitate towards management roles, overseeing several departments or even all medical operations in an establishment.

Healthcare consultant: Building on their expertise, some specialists turn to consultancy, helping other establishments to improve their nuclear medicine practice.

2. Teaching

Professor or lecturer: Those with a passion for imparting knowledge may choose to teach in medical schools or specialist training programmes.

Mentoring and supervision: Acting as a mentor for residents and young professionals is essential to training the next generation of nuclear medicine specialists.

Developing educational programmes: The creation and updating of training programmes in response to developments in nuclear medicine is also crucial.

3. Search

Clinical researcher: Many specialists choose to engage in clinical research, exploring new methods, treatments or technologies in nuclear medicine.

Publications: Writing articles, case studies and reviews is a way of contributing to the medical literature and sharing discoveries with the global medical community.

Interdisciplinary collaboration: The interdisciplinary nature of nuclear medicine offers opportunities for collaboration with other specialities, leading to joint innovations and discoveries.

Career development in nuclear medicine is both stimulating and rewarding. Whether in leadership, education or research, the opportunities are vast and allow professionals to leave a lasting mark on the field. By continuing to learn and adapt, nuclear medicine specialists can continue to have a significant impact on patient health and the advancement of medical science.

Professional networks and dedicated associations.

In the vast field of nuclear medicine, joining a professional network or specialist association is essential for the ongoing exchange of information, continuing education, the defence of professional rights and the sharing of best practice. These associations and networks not only enable us to build relationships, but also to keep abreast of the latest innovations, research studies, technological advances and ethical issues.

1. Worldwide associations
    Société Internationale de Médecine Nucléaire et d'Imagerie Moléculaire (SNMMI): This international organisation aims to promote the exchange of science and education in nuclear medicine.
    World Federation of Nuclear Medicine and Biology (WFNMB): brings together professionals from all over the world and organises conferences, workshops and training courses.
2. Regional and national associations
    European Society of Nuclear Medicine (EANM): plays a crucial role in promoting nuclear medicine in Europe through congresses, publications and clinical guidelines.
    Asian Association of Nuclear Medicine (AOFNMB): Serving the nuclear medicine community in Asia.

National associations: Almost every country has its own nuclear medicine association or society, which deals with issues specific to its region or legislation.

3. Specialty and sub-specialty groups

Associations of nuclear medicine technologists: These associations focus specifically on technologists, who play an essential role in implementing procedures and managing equipment.

Groups dedicated to specific pathologies: For example, groups focusing solely on nuclear cardiology or nuclear oncology.

4. Online forums and networks

Discussion forums: Platforms where professionals can discuss complex cases, share resources or ask for advice.

Social media groups: Groups on platforms such as LinkedIn or Facebook dedicated to nuclear medicine.

Membership of a professional network or association offers many benefits, such as discounts on conferences, access to specialist journals, the opportunity to apply for research grants, and much more. Most importantly, it gives professionals a sense of belonging to a community that is working collectively to improve nuclear medicine and, consequently, patient care.

Chapter 22:
THE EVOLUTION OF THE PROFESSION: LOOKING BACK AND LOOKING FORWARD

Historical development nuclear medicine.

Nuclear medicine, a medical speciality that combines chemistry, physics, biology and medicine, has come an impressive way since its beginnings. Today, it is an invaluable diagnostic and therapeutic tool, using small quantities of radioactive materials to diagnose, assess and treat a variety of diseases. Let's take a look at this exciting journey together.

The origins: Discovery of radioactivity
At the end of the 19th century, scientists began to take an interest in the radiation emanating from certain substances. In 1896, Henri Becquerel discovered radioactivity by studying uranium salts. Shortly afterwards, Pierre and Marie Curie isolated radium and polonium, thus consolidating the study of radioactivity.

The first medical applications
At the beginning of the 20th century, the curative properties of radiation were recognised, particularly in the treatment of tumours. However, their use was primitive and often dangerous, due to a lack of in-depth knowledge.

The advent of artificial isotopes
In 1934, Frédéric and Irène Joliot-Curie succeeded in creating artificial isotopes. This discovery opened the door to the medical use of radioactive isotopes, as they could be specifically designed to emit radiation for a controlled period of time.

The birth of nuclear medicine as a discipline

After the Second World War, with the development of nuclear technology and the increased availability of radioactive isotopes produced by nuclear reactors, medical applications multiplied. The 1950s saw the first thyroid scans using radioactive iodine.

Technological innovations and the development of imaging

The 1960s and 1970s saw the emergence of gamma cameras and computers, enabling the development of scintigraphy as an imaging technique. Positron emission tomography (PET) appeared in the 1980s, offering much higher resolution and the possibility of visualising tissue metabolism.

The era of hybridisation

At the beginning of the 21st century, the combination of PET with computed tomography (CT) enabled functional and anatomical images to be merged, providing a more complete view of pathologies.

Integration with molecular biology

Recently, nuclear medicine has focused on visualising molecular processes within the body, opening up prospects for personalised medicine and targeted therapies.

The history of nuclear medicine is one of convergence between fundamental science and the desire to better understand, diagnose and treat disease. It continues to evolve, with new technological advances and expanding clinical applications, promising an even brighter future for this fascinating discipline.

Major players and pioneers discipline.

Nuclear medicine, like many medical and scientific disciplines, has been shaped by visionary individuals whose determination and ingenuity have pushed back the frontiers of knowledge. Here is a brief introduction to some of the pioneers who have left their mark on the field.

Henri Becquerel (1852-1908): This French physicist laid the foundation stone for nuclear medicine when he discovered radioactivity in 1896, while studying uranium salts. His fundamental discovery paved the way for the many applications of radioactivity in medicine and beyond.

Pierre (1859-1906) and Marie Curie (1867-1934): This famous research couple played a crucial role in isolating and studying radium and polonium. Marie Curie, in particular, was a driving force behind the medical application of radiation, especially during the First World War.

Frédéric (1900-1958) and Irène Joliot-Curie (1897-1956): Continuing the work of Marie and Pierre Curie, this couple succeeded in producing artificial radioactive isotopes in 1934, opening the door to more targeted medical applications.

Benedict Cassen (1902-1972): This biomedical engineer is often credited with developing the first functional gamma camera in 1950. This instrument made it possible to obtain images of the human body after administering radioactive isotopes, thus laying the foundations for scintigraphy.

David E. Kuhl (1929-2017): A pioneer of emission tomography, Kuhl developed the first cross-sectional imaging techniques in the 1960s, preceding the advent of PET by several years.

Hal O. Anger (1920-2005): Often called the "father of the gamma camera", Anger designed and developed the first commercially viable gamma camera in the 1950s, which remains an essential tool in nuclear medicine.

Paul Harper (1921-2008): Harper is credited with introducing the idea of radionuclide therapy, using radioactive isotopes to treat diseases including thyroid cancer.

Each of these pioneers, through their discoveries and innovations, helped to shape nuclear medicine as we know it today. Their work continues to influence and inspire current generations of researchers and clinicians in the field.

Future prospects and challenges for the new generation of nurses.

At the dawn of a new technological era and faced with an ever-changing medical landscape, the new generation of nuclear medicine nurses is faced with a horizon littered with both challenges and tremendous opportunities.

The weight of technological innovation: Technological advances, from robotics to artificial intelligence, promise to transform nuclear medicine. Nurses will have to adapt quickly, acquire new skills and, more than ever, understand the interface between man and machine to guarantee optimal patient care.

Humanising care in a high-tech world: Despite the influx of technology, empathy, listening and compassion remain at the heart of the profession. The challenge will be to maintain this humanity in an increasingly digitised environment, and to remember that behind every image, every piece of data, there is a human being.

New ethical responsibilities: With the power of technology come new ethical concerns. How, for example, should sensitive data be managed? Or how can we ensure fair treatment for all patients in the age of personalised medicine? The new generation of nurses will need to be at the forefront of these debates.

Multidisciplinarity: Nuclear medicine, by its very nature, involves working in close collaboration with other specialities. Interprofessional communication skills and the ability to work in a multidisciplinary team will be more crucial than ever.

The importance of continuing education: Nuclear medicine is evolving rapidly. Nurses will need to devote themselves to training throughout their careers, not only to keep abreast of the latest techniques, but also to anticipate future trends.

Managing stress and mental health: The increasing complexity of care, combined with the pressures of the hospital environment, can take its toll on mental health. Learning how to manage stress, recognise the signs of burn-out and seek help when necessary will be essential.

The globalisation of care: In the age of telemedicine and international collaboration, nurses are likely to have the opportunity to work with patients and professionals from all over the world. Increased cultural sensitivity and an understanding of international medical practices will therefore be essential.

The future looks bright for nuclear medicine, and by extension, for nuclear medicine nurses. While there are many challenges, there are also opportunities to learn, grow and shape the future of this fascinating discipline. By arming the next generation of nurses with the necessary skills, resilience and passion, we can be confident that patient care in nuclear medicine will be in safe hands.

Conclusion

Nuclear medicine :
a constantly evolving field.

Nuclear medicine, a discipline at the crossroads of physics, biology and medicine, has always been the fruit of a constant quest for innovation and improvement. From its modest beginnings in the middle of the 20th century, it has evolved to become one of the pillars of medical diagnosis and treatment, opening up hitherto unexplored horizons.

The basic principle of nuclear medicine is based on the use of radioactive substances, known as radiopharmaceuticals, to visualise, diagnose and even treat certain diseases. What began with simple images has evolved into sophisticated imaging techniques such as positron emission tomography (PET) or scintigraphy, capable of providing detailed images of the body's metabolic processes.

Technological developments have been the driving force behind this discipline. For example, modern PET-CT machines combine PET with computed tomography (CT), allowing more accurate visualisation of metabolic abnormalities by superimposing them on anatomical structure. This has been a revolutionary change for the detection and management of various conditions, including cancers.

But nuclear medicine does not stop at simple imaging. It has broadened its spectrum to include treatments such as targeted internal radiotherapy. In these protocols, specific radiopharmaceuticals target the diseased cells, enabling selective destruction while sparing the surrounding healthy tissue.

Ethical and environmental challenges have also influenced this discipline. Faced with growing concern about radiation exposure, techniques have been perfected to minimise doses while maximising clinical benefits. Similarly, responsible management of radioactive waste has become an absolute priority.

The development of nuclear medicine has also been marked by interdisciplinary collaboration. Radiopharmacists, medical physicists, doctors and technologists work closely together to improve existing techniques and develop new ones. This synergy is essential if we are to push the boundaries of what this discipline can achieve.

Looking to the future, nuclear medicine is poised to embrace artificial intelligence and big data, with the hope of further personalising treatments and improving diagnostic accuracy. Advances in genomics and molecular biology could also pave the way for even more targeted therapies.

Nuclear medicine, which is constantly evolving, embodies the fusion of science and medicine, always on the lookout for new ways to improve patients' lives. In a world where technology and medicine are coming ever closer together, this discipline is set to play a decisive role in the medical landscape of the 21st century.

The nurse :
an essential pillar of patient care.

At the heart of healthcare systems, nurses play an essential and versatile role in the overall care of patients. Much more than simply performing technical tasks, nurses are the key players in ensuring the continuity, quality and safety of care. With their clinical expertise, ability to listen and patient-centred approach, nurses are undeniably an essential pillar of care.

As soon as patients are admitted, it is often the nurse who becomes their first point of contact, assessing their needs, reassuring them and establishing a relationship of trust. This therapeutic relationship is at the heart of the nursing profession. It fosters communication, facilitates understanding of treatment and supports patients throughout their care.

In addition to their clinical skills, nurses play a crucial role in coordinating care. They work with a multitude of healthcare professionals - doctors, pharmacists, care assistants, social workers, psychologists and many others - to ensure holistic patient care. They act as the link between these different players, ensuring that essential information is passed on and that the patient receives coherent, comprehensive care.

Nurses' educational skills are also essential. They are often the ones who educate patients and their families about the disease, the treatments, the possible side-effects, and the daily routine to be adopted. This educational aspect is vital in enabling patients to take charge of their own health, understand and adhere to their treatments, and optimise their autonomy.

But the nurse's role does not stop there. Their proximity to the patient puts them on the front line in detecting changes in the patient's state of health, anticipating complications or assessing the patient's pain and comfort. Their sharp eye, combined with their clinical expertise, makes them the true guardians of patient safety.

Furthermore, humanity and empathy are at the heart of the nursing profession. At times of vulnerability, pain, or in the face of the unknown, the emotional support provided by the nurse is just as essential as the technical care. They comfort, listen and understand, accompanying patients through the ups and downs of their care.

Nurses are much more than just those who carry out tasks. They are the guardians of quality care, the defenders of patients' interests, and the link between all those involved in healthcare. In an ever-changing medical world, where technology plays an increasingly important role, the human, close and caring role of the nurse remains, more than ever, an essential pillar of patient care.

Glossary of specific medical terms.

Scintigraphy: Imaging technique that uses radioactive isotopes to visualise the activity of an organ or region of the body.

PET (Positron Emission Tomography): Imaging technique that measures the metabolic activity of tissues using radioactive tracers.

Gamma camera: Device used to detect the radiation emitted by radioactive isotopes introduced into the body.

Radiopharmaceutical: Radioactive substance used in nuclear medicine for diagnosis or treatment.

Radioactive isotope: A variant of a chemical element that emits radiation in the form of particles or rays.

Radiation: Energy emitted in the form of waves or particles.

Radiation protection: A set of measures designed to protect individuals and the environment against the harmful effects of radiation.

Radioactive dose: Quantity of radioactivity administered or received by a patient or organ.

Stochastic effects: Effects whose probability of occurrence increases with the dose, but whose severity does not depend on the dose (e.g. cancer).

Deterministic effects: Effects whose severity increases with dose, and which require a minimum dose to manifest themselves (e.g. radiation burns).

Ionising radiation : Radiation that has enough energy to detach electrons from atoms or molecules, which can damage or kill cells.

PET-CT (Positron Emission Tomography - Computed Tomography): Combination of PET with computed tomography (CT) to obtain functional and anatomical images in a single session.

Dosimetry: Science that measures the amount of radiation absorbed by a material or tissue.

Biodistribution: Distribution of a substance, such as a radiopharmaceutical, through the different tissues of the body.

Radiology: Branch of medicine that uses radiation to diagnose and treat disease.

Telemedicine: the practice of medicine at a distance using information and communication technologies.

Onco-haematology: Medical speciality dedicated to the study and treatment of cancers and blood diseases.

Radiotoxicity: Toxicity resulting from exposure to ionising radiation.

Radionuclide therapy: Treatment that uses radionuclides to deliver radiation directly to a tumour or a specific area of the body.

This glossary provides an overview of some of the key terms associated with nuclear medicine and radiology. For clinical or academic use, a more comprehensive glossary and additional sources may be required.

Additional resources and recommendations for continuing education.

Books and Manuals:
> "Essentials of Nuclear Medicine Imaging" by Fred A. Mettler and Milton J. Guiberteau.
>
> "Nuclear Medicine: The Requisites" by Harvey A. Ziessman, Janis P. O'Malley and James H. Thrall.

Specialist journals:
> Journal of Nuclear Medicine (JNM)
>
> European Journal of Nuclear Medicine and Molecular Imaging
>
> Seminars in Nuclear Medicine

Associations and companies:
> Society of Nuclear Medicine and Molecular Imaging (SNMMI)
>
> European Association of Nuclear Medicine (EANM)
>
> International Atomic Energy Agency (IAEA) - Nuclear medicine section

Online training and webinars:
> SNMMI Learning Center: Offers courses, webinars and online seminars for professionals.
>
> EANM e-Learning: Online training platform for nuclear medicine professionals.

Conferences and workshops:
> Annual conferences organised by SNMMI, EANM and other relevant associations.
>
> Practical workshops on specific subjects such as dosimetry, the use of new cameras and radiation risk management.

Certification programmes and post-graduate training:

Specialist certification in nuclear medicine for nurses, technicians and doctors.

Nuclear medicine residency programmes for doctors.

Online resources:

Radiopaedia: A collaborative reference site for radiology, which also includes a section on nuclear medicine.

Medscape: A platform for healthcare professionals with articles, case studies and news in the field of nuclear medicine.

Interdisciplinary collaboration networks:

Forums and discussion groups dedicated to nuclear medicine.

Collaboration with foreign c e n t r e s t o exchange knowledge and practices.

Regulatory bodies and standards:

To keep abreast of standards and regulations, it is advisable to follow the publications of the IAEA and national health authorities.

Technology watch:

Keeping abreast of technological advances via specialist magazines, newsletters and exhibitions at conferences.

Books and Manuals:

"Manuel de médecine nucléaire" by Jean-Noël Talbot.

"Atlas de scintigraphie osseuse" by Françoise Montravers.

Specialist journals:

Nuclear Medicine - Functional and metabolic imaging

Revue Française des Laboratoires

Associations and companies:

- French Society of Nuclear Medicine and Molecular Imaging (SFMN)
- Canadian Association of Nuclear Medicine (CANM)

Online training and webinars:
- The SFMN and ACMN websites often offer training courses, online seminars and webinars for professionals.

Conferences and workshops:
- Annual conferences organised by SFMN, ACMN and other relevant French-speaking associations.
- Specialist workshops are offered at these meetings.

Certification programmes and post-graduate training:
- University and inter-university diplomas specific to nuclear medicine offered by various French-speaking universities.

Online resources:
- Campus numérique en radiologie (CAMPUS R3): French-language platform offering teaching modules in medical imaging, including nuclear medicine.

Interdisciplinary collaboration networks:
- French-speaking forums and discussion groups specialising in nuclear medicine.

Regulatory bodies and standards:
- Autorité de Sûreté Nucléaire (ASN) for France: regulates, among other things, medical practices using radionuclides.

Technology watch:
- To keep abreast of technological advances and new techniques, the SFMN and ACMN newsletters and equipment supplier publications are excellent resources.

It is essential for nuclear medicine professionals to continue their training. Not only to guarantee the quality of their care, but also to remain at the cutting edge of a constantly evolving discipline. Although there are sometimes fewer resources available in French than in English, they are of a high quality and tailored to the specific needs of each country.